Herbal Medicine: A Concise Overview for Professionals

Edited by

Professor Edzard Ernst MD, PhD FRCP (Edin)
Department of Complementary Medicine
School of Postgraduate Medicine and Health Sciences,
University of Exeter, UK

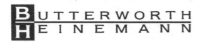
BUTTERWORTH
HEINEMANN

OXFORD   AUCKLAND   BOSTON   JOHANNESBURG   MELBOURNE   NEW DELHI

Butterworth-Heinemann
Linacre House, Jordan Hill, Oxford OX2 8DP
225 Wildwood Avenue, Woburn, MA 01801-2041
A division of Reed Educational and Professional Publishing Ltd

Ⓡ A member of the Reed Elsevier plc group

First published 2000

British Library Cataloguing in Publication Data
Herbal medicine: a concise overview for professionals
   1. Herbs — Therapeutic use
   I. Ernst, E., 1948–
   615.3'21

   ISBN 0 7506 4540 7

Library of Congress Cataloguing in Publication Data
A catalogue record for this book is available from the Library of Congress

ISBN 0 7506 4540 7

Typeset by Bath Typesetting
Printed and bound in Great Britain by Biddles Ltd, Guildford and King's Lynn

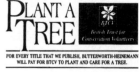

Contents

Contributors

L. A. Anderson BPharm PhD MRPharmS
Principal Pharmaceutical Officer, Medicines Control Agency, Market Towers, 1 Nine Elms Lane, Vauxhall, London, UK

J. Barnes BPharm MRPharmS
Research Fellow, Centre for Pharmacognosy & Phytotherapy, School of Pharmacy, University of London, 29–39 Brunswick Square, London, UK

E. Ernst MD PhD FRCP (Edin)
Director, Department of Complementary Medicine, School of Postgraduate Medicine and Health Sciences, University of Exeter, 25 Victoria Park Road, Exeter, UK

S. B. A. Halkes PhD
Post-Doc Research Associate, Department of Medicinal Chemistry, Faculty of Pharmacy, Universiteit Utrecht, PO Box 80082, 3508 TB Utrecht, The Netherlands

P. J. Houghton BPharm PhD FRPharmS CChem FRSC
Department of Pharmacy, King's College, London, UK

D. Loew Prof. Dr. Med
Institute of Clinical Pharmacology, University of Frankfurt, Theodor Stern-Kai 7, 60590 Frankfurt, Germany

L. Milner BA FSA
Laurel House, Corbridge, Northumberland, UK

E. K. Perry BSc PhD DSc
MRC Neurochemical Unit, Newcastle General Hospital, Newcastle upon Tyne, UK

M. H. Pittler, MD
Department of Complementary Medicine, School of Postgraduate
Medicine and Health Sciences, University of Exeter, 25 Victoria Park
Road, Exeter, UK

A. Schroedter Dr.
Department of Clinical Pharmacology, University of Frankfurt,
Theodor Stern-Kai 7, 60590 Frankfurt, Germany

H. Wagner Prof. Dr.
Centre of Pharma-Research, Pharmaceutical Biology, University of
Munich, Butenandtstr. 5, 81377 Munich, Germany

E. M. Williamson BSc PhD MRPharmS FLS
Lecturer in Pharmacognosy, Centre for Pharmacognosy, The School
of Pharmacy, University of London, 29/39 Brunswick Square,
London, UK

Preface

With the advent of modern synthetic drugs about 100 years ago, herbal medicine ceased to be the mainstay of therapeutics. In some countries, for example the UK and the USA, this process rendered medical herbalism almost extinct. In other countries, such as Germany, medical herbalism continued to play a role but was pushed somewhat towards the fringe of mainstream medicine.

Today medical herbalism is back in the limelight. In fact, it is more popular than ever before, and sales figures in some countries (for example the USA) are booming beyond the wildest expectations of the manufacturers. The reasons for its renaissance are complex, but clearly have to be considered in connection with what could be described as the 'greening of medicine'. The *Zeitgeist* of the dawning millennium has become strongly in favour of all things natural. Natural, we are led to believe, is safe, ecological and in tune with nature. Frequently, consumers don't seem to question these somewhat naïve assumptions.

In parallel with the consumers' vote in favour of plant-based medicines, and in many ways driven by this force, medical herbalism has gradually changed into what may be called rational phytomedicine. Over many years, plant pharmacologists and other scientists have accumulated a wealth of knowledge on the chemical constituents of plants and their pharmacological actions. With much more hesitation and considerable delay, clinicians have begun to test herbal remedies in rigorous clinical trials. These activities have largely been confined to the European continent, but are now spreading to other countries as well. By applying the rules of science, traditional herbalism is now being transformed into science-based phytomedicine.

In the USA, where the 'herbal boom' of the recent years has been most impressive, and also in other countries, urgent questions are emerging:

- How efficacious are these remedies?
- How do phytomedicines work?
- What can we learn from traditional herbalism?
- What are the adverse effects of these medicines, and how can we minimize them?
- How should the quality of herbal medicines be standardized?
- How should phytomedicines be regulated?
- How should future research strategies be designed?

This book cannot offer all the answers. It does, however, point the reader in the right direction. It represents an attempt to give a balanced introduction and provide access to the relatively new world of rational phytomedicine. It is written by some of the leading experts in phytomedicine worldwide, who summarize the present state of the art in a clearly structured, scientific way. Its approach is strictly evidence-based. We are confident that this volume fulfils an urgent need and will prove to be a valuable addition to the English medical literature.

The book aims to serve as a useful, fully referenced guide for physicians, medical herbalists and other healthcare professionals with an interest in plant-based therapy. It is also relevant for healthcare policy makers, manufacturers of herbal products and medical educators. I hope readers will be content with our efforts to supply a concise introductory text to scientific phytomedicine and modern medical herbalism.

E. Ernst
Exeter, June 1999

1

From ancient texts to modern phytotherapy: plants in mind

E. K. Perry, L. Milner and P. J. Houghton

Introduction

It is common knowledge in many of today's societies that plants or their extracts continue to provide effective treatment for diseases of all kind, as they have done for centuries. Ayurvedic medicine in India and traditional Chinese medicine both depend, to a large extent, on the use of precise plant-based prescriptions for the treatment of specific disorders. Similar contemporary practices are to be found in many regions – for example in other parts of Asia, in South America, Africa, the Middle East and Russia. Western medicine, in contrast, largely abandoned medicines based on plant extracts in favour of the use of isolated or synthetic single chemicals. The perceived advantage of dose control was consistent with prevailing reductionist scientific models and with commercial incentives associated with the patenting of novel chemicals as drugs. Surprisingly, many professional and lay individuals in the West today have no idea that plants have provided, still provide or could provide useful medicines. Such a concept is often relegated to the realms of 'alternative' or 'complementary' medicine and considered to be no more than quaint but irrelevant folklore. At the beginning of the twenty-first century, however, there is a turning of the tide; a trend that could be described as 'back to the future', with increasing numbers of contemporary scientists and medical practitioners considering plants and their chemicals as sources of novel, effective and safer drugs. One of the key events that eventually triggered this paradigm shift was the tragedy of birth defects induced by the anti-emetic synthetic chemical thalidomide. Since then, safety issues concerning current pharmacotherapies have dominated the minds of an increasing proportion of the Western population. Whilst plant-based drugs can be as toxic as any synthetic chemical if improperly used, there is the advantage that where the former have been employed for hundreds or even thousands of years, such medicines have been extensively tried, tested and appraised. Moreover, it is not unlikely that evolution has played some role in generating mechanisms in animals, including man, for exploiting plants to promote health beyond nutritional needs.

This chapter focuses on drugs affecting the nervous system, and provides some examples of plant chemicals currently used in orthodox Western medicine that are of ethnic origin and have since gained scientific credibility in terms of pharmacological mechanisms (chemicals from plants such as the opium poppy, coca bush and belladonna). A discussion of some of the plants/plant chemicals emerging from the realms of alternative or complementary medicine into the field of modern science for the treatment of such disorders as Alzheimer's, Parkinson's disease and depression follows. These provide examples of the potential, still largely unexplored in modern pharmacology, to select promising plant species from archival or ethnic sources and investigate their biological activity and clinical efficacy in the context of current biological models.

Plant chemicals (or derivatives) established in modern medicine

John Mann, in his fascinating book *Murder, Magic and Medicine* (Mann, 1992), provides a detailed description of the use of the opium poppy (*Papaver somniferum*) by the Sumerians (4000 BC), ancient Greeks and Romans to relieve pain and induce sleep. The use of extracts (e.g. laudanum) for this purpose continued through to the twentieth century, during the first half of which the chemical structure of morphine was identified, and during the second half of which two major discoveries about the brain were made. The existence in the brain of receptor molecules that bind chemicals from the opium poppy (such as morphine), the so-called opiate receptors, was described by Pert and Snyder in 1973. This raised the question of whether the brain makes its own analgesic chemicals. These chemicals were discovered shortly after by Hughes *et al.*, (1975), who isolated enkephalin peptides from the brain; these bound to the opiate receptors and elicited analgesia.

Other important drugs that owe their discovery to ancient practices include cocaine and derivative alkaloids from the coca bush (*Erythroxylum coca*) and the tropane alkaloids scopolamine and atropine from the Solanaceae plant family. Coca leaves have been and still are used by South American Indians to sustain energy and physical activity – for example, in the remarkable feat of erecting buildings (such as those of the Incas) at very high altitudes (Karch, 1997). Cocaine blocks ion channels, and one of its actions is to inhibit the re-uptake of dopamine and noradrenaline in the brain, thus accounting for its invigorating effects. Another aspect of the sustaining properties of coca leaves is a numbing of the senses. Although Sigmund Freud – notorious as an advocate of the recreational use of cocaine – noted the numbing effects of the drug on the tongue, it was only later that the drug was discovered by Carl Köller in 1884 to function as a local anaesthetic (see Mann, 1992), with derivatives such as procaine and lidocaine becoming the mainstay of local anaesthesia.

Plants belonging to the Solanaceae family include mandrake (*Mandragora officinarum*) and belladonna (*Atropa belladona*), which have a long history in ritualistic/religious practices where alterations in consciousness (e.g. hallucinations) are induced (Perry and Perry, 1995). Less well known is the use of these plants to reduce awareness of pain and induce sleep. Dioscorides, a Greek physician to the Roman army at the beginning of the first millennium, recorded in his *Materia Medica* the use of mandrake to induce sleep during surgery. In modern anaesthesia scopolamine, which together with atropine is one of the main alkaloids in this and related species, has been used until recently to induce 'twilight sleep' during childbirth, in which the patient is awake but not aware of or able to recall the experience. Other plants of this family, such as henbane (*Hyoscyamus niger*) and datura (*Datura stramonium*), have also been used in ancient Greek and American Shamanic rituals to induce 'madness' and prophecy (Schultes and Hofmann, 1992). This 'model' of madness is consistent with current understanding of the mechanisms of dementia (Perry, 1997), since atropine and scopolamine block the action of the brain transmitter signal, acetylcholine, on cholinergic muscarinic receptors. In diseases like Alzheimer's this transmitter is lost, and new synthetic drugs are being prescribed to rectify the loss.

Phytochemicals for the treatment of Alzheimer's disease

Ancient texts

While newly introduced synthetic cholinesterase inhibitors such as tacrine (Cognex), donepezil (Aricept) or rivastigmine (Exelon) provide a minority of patients with some symptomatic relief, most patients with Alzheimer's disease have not yet benefited substantially from the major financial investments in Western scientific research and drug development programmes. Ethnobotanical evidence derived from cultural, empirical or complementary medical uses of plants can be examined for new directions in therapeutic research strategies.

European use of plant products in this context may be more widespread than is appreciated by orthodox medical practitioners. Rosemary (*Rosmarinus officinalis*), for example, is used by practising medical herbalists and aromatherapists in the United Kingdom for memory problems (Price and Price, 1995; Bartram, 1995). *Ginkgo biloba*, popular because of its perceived anti-ageing properties, including enhancing cerebral activity (Kleijnen and Knipschild, 1992; Vesper and Hadgen, 1994), has recently been reported to be of therapeutic value in mild to moderately affected patients with Alzheimer's disease (Burkard and Lehri, 1991; Kanowski *et al.*, 1996; Le Bars *et al.*, 1997). In the 1997 placebo-controlled, double-blind, randomized trial, the standardized *Ginkgo biloba* extract EG6761 was associated with significant improvements in cognitive function (ADAS-Cog) and caregivers' rating (GERRI) when compared with placebo. Equally importantly, there were no significant differences in the number, incidence or severity of adverse side effects. There are numerous other documented (although more anecdotal) examples of cognitive-enhancing plants in non-Westernized societies. These include components of traditional Chinese herbal prescriptions like FuQuiDiHuang, Indian Ayurvedic medicines (Manyam, 1999) and plants used by Northwest Amazon Indians (Schultes, 1993). In Western societies, which have abandoned plant medicines, such evidence is based on old texts. In his introduction to John Riddle's (1985) historical analysis of the contribution of the Greek physician Pedanios Dioscorides to pharmacy and medicine, John Scarborough states that: 'One must command the ancient texts in their original tongues and one must use modern pharmacognosy in judicious association with the ancient data'.

In selecting texts for information on the historical use of plant medicines, it is important to focus on the most relevant cultures. The ancient Greeks, for example, took a dim view of ageing. According to Pythagoras (seventh century BC): 'The scene of mortal existence closes, after a great length of time to which fortunately few of the human species arrives. The system returns to the imbecility of the first epoch of infancy' (Halpert, 1983). Aristotle (383–322 BC) was also convinced that old age is inseparable from mental failure, asserting that: 'There is not much left of the acumen of the mind which helped them in their youth, nor of the faculties which served the intellect (imagination, power of reasoning and memory)' (Halpert, 1983). The Romans, however, were more optimistic, and Cicero (second century BC) stated that: 'It is our duty to resist old age; to compensate for its deficits by a watchful care; to fight against it as we would fight against disease. Much greater care is due to the mind and soul, for they, too, like lamps grow dim with time unless we supply them with oil' (Mahendra, 1987).

In medieval times, records relating to prominent individuals indicate that life-spans of 70–90 years were not uncommon, and in one thirteenth century medical Cambridge text it was noted that: 'Anyone is likely from time to time to lose their memory and their senses. If they do not have immediate help, this could result in death. Take marigold and southernwood and do not forget sage whoever wants to recover his memory should include in his diet those herbs I have listed above' (Hunt, 1990).

A recent search through some of the medical herbals published over the last centuries has provided interesting information on plants that might be worth investigating in relation to dementia therapy (Perry *et al.*, 1998). Between the sixteenth and eighteenth centuries, several plants acquired a persistent reputation for memory-enhancing properties. It was, for example, noted about balm (*Melissa officinalis*) that: 'An essence of balm, given in canary wine, every morning will renew youth, strengthen the brain' (*London Dispensary*, 1696), and that: 'Balm is sovereign for the brain, strengthening the memory and powerfully chasing away the melancholy (Evelyn, 1699). Paracelsus believed it would completely revivify a man, and it was formerly esteemed of great use in all complaints supposed to proceed from a disordered state of the nervous system (Grieve, 1931). Thomas Coghan also recommended in 1584 that balm tea should be consumed daily by his students to help clear the head, increase understanding and sharpen the memory. These statements obtain a degree of support from a recent report of a placebo-controlled assessment of the effects of aromatherapy using balm essential oil (combined with lavender). A small number of patients with dementia were reported to improve on measures of independence and general functioning in comparison with those exposed to a culinary vegetable oil (Mitchell, 1993). It may be of particular interest that balm, in addition to its reputation for memory enhancement, is also widely known for its ability to reduce restlessness and agitation (Grieve, 1931; Bartram, 1995). The effects in Alzheimer's disease are not confined to impairing memory, but also involve behavioural changes such as agitation and wandering, which are as much in need of treatment as cognitive dysfunction.

Sage (*Salvia officinalis*), another member of the Labiatae plant family, also had a reputation for memory enhancement to judge from the following sixteenth to eighteenth century texts (see also above): 'It is singularly good for the head and brain and quickenethe the nerves and memory' (Gerard, 1597); 'It also heals the memory, warming and quickening the senses' (Culpeper, 1652); 'Because it is good against palsies and comforts the sinews and brain it must needs be good for students (Coghan, 1584); 'Sage will retard that rapid progress of decay that treads upon our heels so fast in latter years of life, will preserve faculty and memory more valuable to the rational mind than life itself' (Hill, 1755). Sage species are also used in Ayurvedic medicine, one of the longest established and still practised forms of herbal medicine, 'to clear emotional obstructions from the mind and for promoting calmness and clarity' (McIntyre, 1996). In traditional Chinese medicine, *Nao Li Kang* (which translates as 'restore brain power granules') contains four ingredients, one of which is a species of sage, and is reported to be effective in 40 per cent of Alzheimer patients (Fu and Fruehof, 1995). The independent use of the same plant genus for a common clinical effect in such widely differing cultures in India, China and Europe is impressive. Sage, while still to be tested in controlled trials, has bioactivities relevant to mechanisms disrupted in Alzheimer's disease.

Consistent with current aromatherapeutic application of rosemary to improve memory, this herb was considered by the ancient Greeks to stimulate the mind, in particular memory (Le Strange, 1977), and students then used to wear sprigs or garlands of the plant as an aide-memoire. According to Roger Hacket, a Doctor of Divinity in 1607 (Grieve, 1931): 'It helpeth the brain, strengtheneth the memorie and is very medicinable for the head'. In the *Grete Herball* (1526), it was recorded that: 'Against weyknesse of the brayne and coldness thereof, sethe rosmaria in wyne and late the pacyent receye the smoke at his nose' (cited in Grieve, 1931). Gerard noted in 1597 that: 'Rosemary comforteth the braine, the memorie, the inward sense'. In *Hamlet*, written in 1601 by William Shakespeare, who was a neighbour of John Gerard, Ophelia said 'There's rosemary; that's for remembrance. Pray, love, remember'. Whether rosemary is of value in treating memory loss in old age, as occurs in Alzheimer's disease, remains to be established by controlled trials and relevant pharmacological research.

It is intriguing to consider how the opinions expressed in these old herbal encyclopaedias originated, whether mainly on the basis of subjective experience, independently, or originating from a common historical source. However, such archival evidence may provide clues for new drug development as valuable as evidence from contemporary non-Western societies when examined in the context of current models of dementia such as Alzheimer's disease.

Modern phytochemistry and pharmacology

For natural plant products to be incorporated into mainstream medicine, both clinical efficacy and relevant biological activity need to be demonstrated. In Alzheimer's disease, potential therapeutic targets in terms of biological mechanisms include:

- Enhancing cholinergic transmission, restricting oxidative stress and inflammatory reactions
- Preventing β-amyloid formation or toxicity
- Elevating circulating oestrogen and levels of other neurotrophic agents such as nerve growth factor.

To date, only cholinergic agents, specifically inhibitors of the enzyme acetylcholinesterase, have been licensed for treatment. Evidence exists for relevant bioactivities in some of the plants mentioned above. There is, for example, a substantial literature on relevant properties of ginkgolides, the chemical constituents of *Ginkgo biloba* considered to be responsible for the medicinal effects of the plant. Specific ginkgolides interact with the cholinergic system (Taylor, 1986) and have neuroprotective or regenerative activities (Bruno *et al.*, 1993; Smith *et al.*, 1996). Any or all of these are potentially relevant to efficacy in dementia therapy. In addition, flavonoids present in *Ginkgo biloba* have antioxidant properties.

Several other traditional Chinese medicinal herb extracts or chemicals have also been investigated for their effects in current dementia models. For example, peony (*Paeonia suffruticosa*) is a component of traditional Chinese herbal prescriptions for dementia, such as Jin Gui Shen Qi Wen, which include Liu Wei Ki Huang Wan. A major chemical constituent of this plant, paeoniflorin, improves radial maze performance in rats impaired by cholinergic blocking agents such as scopolamine (Ohta *et al.*, 1993). Liu Wei Di Huang Wan (Hachimi-jio-gan in Japanese), a mixture of plants also containing peony, is anti-amnesic in this model and increases cortical cholinergic activity (Hirokawa *et al.*, 1996). Shimotus-to, another plant mixture also active in this animal model (Watanabe *et al.*, 1991), contains both peony and Japanese angelica (*Angelica sinensis*) root. The latter species also reverses scopolamine-induced performance deficits (Ohta *et al.*, 1993), and it would be interesting to establish if it is chemically closely related to the European species of angelica, *Angelica archangelica*, which contains nicotinic activity (Wren, 1985; Perry N. *et al.*, 1996).

Cholinesterase inhibitors have been chemically identified in several traditional Chinese medicinal plants, including *Angelica sinensis* and *Evodia rutaecarpa* (Park *et al.*, 1996). Another plant cholinesterase inhibitor, huperzine A, derived from the moss *Huperzia serrata* and traditionally used to treat not only inflammation and fever but also age-related changes in mental function (Houghton, 1999), is currently used in Alzheimer's disease therapy in China (Cheng *et al.*, 1996; Cheng and Tang, 1998; Skolnick, 1997). It is a relatively selective inhibitor of cortical and hippocampal cholinesterase and of acetyl, compared to butyrylcholinesterase. In placebo-controlled randomized trials, huperzine is significantly better than placebo in improving memory, cognition and behavioural function (Xu *et al.*, 1995).

The Ayurvedic herbal formulation Mentat (which consists of 26 plant species) reverses scopolamine-induced memory impairment in animal models (Battacharia *et al.*, 1995). Trasina (five plant species) also reverses memory impairments associated with surgical lesions of the cholinergic basal forebrain (Bhattacharia and Kumar, 1997). Systemic administration of *Withania somnifera* (Indian ginseng), reputed in India to attenuate cerebral deficits including amnesia, led to differential inhibition of acetylcholinesterase and enhanced M1-muscarinic receptor binding in rat brain (Schliebs *et al.*, 1997). Korean ginseng (*Panax ginseng*) is, among other numerous beneficial effects, considered to improve memory (Reid, 1986), and has also been reported to enhance cholinergic activity in similar animal models (Nitta *et al.*, 1995; Salim *et al.*, 1997), to have neuroprotective effects *in vitro* (Wen *et al.*, 1996; Lim *et al.*, 1997) and to interact with nicotinic cholinergic receptors (Lewis *et al.*, 1999).

Among some of the European plant species identified above, there is also evidence of bioactivities relevant to memory function. Balm contains various monoterpenes such as citral and citronella, which have been reported to concentrate in the hippocampus (Mills, 1993) – a key area concerned with learning affected at an early stage by Alzheimer-type pathology (e.g. plaques and tangles). Examining the *in vitro* effects of crude plant extracts of sage and balm on human brain acetylcholinesterase, dose-dependent inhibitory effects on the enzyme (with IC_{50} values of $< 0.1 \mu l$ essential oil per ml) were identified (Perry N. *et al.*, 1996). Several different sources and species of Salvia had similar effects, suggesting that one or more of its chemical constituents are active. *Salvia officinalis* is potentially toxic in high doses on account of its thujone content (Wren, 1985). However, thujone is not present in significant amounts in *Salvia lavandulaefolia* (Spanish sage), which had equally potent inhibitory effects on the enzyme (Perry N. *et al.*, 1996). The active constituents are likely to be other monoterpenoids, which inhibit acetylcholines-terase, albeit at relatively high concentrations (Miyazawa *et al.*, 1997; Perry N. *et al.*, 1999a), and there is evidence of synergy such that inhibitory effects of the essential oil are greater than those of the sum of the active constituent terpenes (Perry N. *et al.*, 1999a). Sage may well be a 'wise remedy', and clinical trials of this species are being initiated in view of its cholinergic and other documented (oestrogenic, antioxidant and anti-inflammatory) properties (Perry N. *et al.*, 1999b) relevant to the treatment of the ageing brain and on account of the archival clinical evidence discussed above. Not only synergistic but also 'polypharmacological' effects are common in the practice of medical herbalism.

In addition to inhibitory effects on brain acetylcholinesterase, balm leaf extracts also interacted with the nicotinic cholinergic receptor, inhibiting (^{3}H)-nicotine binding in a dose-dependent fashion (Perry N. *et al.*, 1996; Wake *et al.*, 1999). Direct stimulation of the nicotinic receptor is likely to be a valid therapeutic approach. This receptor was originally classified on the basis of its interaction with nicotine, the principal alkaloid derived from tobacco (*Nicotiana tabacum*). Since its original introduction into Europe as a treatment for headache (Matthee, 1995), numerous medicinal uses of tobacco have been claimed – for dropsy, epilepsy, malaria, hernia, insomnia, constipation and even hiccoughs. In 1659, Dr Giles Everard recorded that 'to strengthen the memory, the smoke is excellent taken by the nostrils'. Current epidemiological and clinical (e.g. cognitive-enhancing) evidence of the potential value of nicotine in Alzheimer's therapy (reviewed by Court and Perry, 1994) may thus have some precedent in traditional medical usage. Nicotine is now known to enhance memory and attention in animal models and in human volunteers. The risk of developing Alzheimer's disease is, on average, halved in tobacco smokers (Lee, 1994), although this evidence remains controversial. Nicotine is also protective in a variety of models associated with ischaemic, β-amyloid peptide and glutamate toxicity (Clementi *et al.*, 1999). There are significantly fewer β-amyloid plaques in the brains of tobacco smokers compared with non-smokers (Ulrich *et al.*, 1997; Court *et al.*, 1998). Despite such evidence supporting the use of nicotine to prevent brain ageing, nicotine is a potentially toxic alkaloid with adverse cardiovascular and gastrointestinal effects. If other nicotinic chemicals with a different structure exist in plant species reputed to enhance memory, their therapeutic value may be greater.

It is not unexpected to discover novel cholinergic activities in plants. Endogenous cholinergic chemicals deter animal predators of the plant by interacting with peripheral and/or central cholinergic systems, impairing physiological functions at higher concentrations. A variety of cholinergic phytochemicals such as physostigmine, huperzine and galanthamine have already been identified (Perry *et al.*, 1998) and further chemicals with cholinergic activity continue to be discovered; for example berberine in corydalis tuber (Hwang *et al.*, 1996). These chemicals are alkaloids (nitrogen-containing secondary metabolites) that are without exception toxic at low concentrations, and the plants from which they are derived generally belong to the category of known poisonous species. Their therapeutic value is thus restricted in terms of dosage and chronic applications. Preventative, protective and symptomatic strategies in a progressive, degenerative disease such as Alzheimer's are likely to involve long-term application. Species such as Salvia or Melissa, noted in ancient texts to improve mental function, are not considered poisonous unless at a very high dosage. Cholinergic activities in these species can be presumed, if alkaloid, to be present in very low concentrations. Other types of secondary plant metabolites, such as volatile terpenes (the principal constituents of essential oils, some of which inhibit acetylcholinesterase) present in many Labiatae species (which include sage and balm), are more likely to attract animals (e.g. insect pollinators). There may be greater therapeutic value, at least in terms of safety, in plant products that evolved to attract rather than repel animal (including human) species. Exactly how such terpenoids interact with neurons is not yet established, although in addition to enzyme inhibition, interaction of a terpene (cembranox) with the nicotinic receptor has been recently reported (Hann *et al.*, 1998).

Comparisons with 'rational' therapies

Some of the examples provided indicate the potential of a combined ethnobotanical and pharmacognostical approach to developing therapies in the treatment of Alzheimer's disease. Current orthodox Western strategies in dementia therapy, however rationally based, are not all consistent with cultural traditions. Physostygmine, for example, the prototypic cholinesterase inhibitor whose short half-life *in vivo* led to the search for longer-acting inhibitors, is not renowned for its traditional uses in memory enhancement. *Physostigma venonosa*, the calabar bean, found in West Africa, was used locally as an emetic in trials of witchcraft by ordeal (Mann, 1992). The synthetic inhibitor tacrine was originally used to recover consciousness in cases of drug overdose (e.g. of antidepressants with antimuscarinic actions). Galanthamine, a longer-acting naturally-occurring enzyme inhibitor derived from the bulbs of *Galanthus nivalis* (snowdrop) or *Narcissus* (daffodil), provides significant clinical benefit in patients with Alzheimer's disease, although adverse effects include nausea and vomiting (Fulton and Benfield, 1996). Grieve (1931) records the use of daffodils as an emetic, antidote to poisons and for external use. None of the encyclopaedias mentions the use of this species for memory enhancement. Interestingly, both physo-stigmine and galanthamine, in addition to being cholinesterase inhibitors, are also non-competitive nicotinic channel activators (Pereira *et al.*, 1993), which may be of added value in Alzheimer's therapy (above).

Phytochemicals for the treatment of other central nervous system disorders

Depression

The publication in the *British Medical Journal* (Linde *et al.*, 1996) of the results of a systematic review and meta-analysis of clinical trials of St John's wort (*Hypericum perforatum*) for the treatment of depression was a landmark in 'border crossing' between alternative and orthodox medical paradigms. In 23 randomized trials, including a total of 1757 outpatients with mild or moderately severe depression (15 placebo-controlled trials and eight comparing St John's wort with other drug treatments), hypericum extracts were found to be significantly superior to control by a factor of 2.7, and as effective as standard antidepressants. Although most readily accessible herbals refer to more general use of the plant (e.g. wound-healing), Culpeper recorded its use 'against melancholy and madness'.

Brain mechanisms underlying depression are not yet fully understood, but are considered to involve disturbances in mono-aminergic transmitter systems such as serotonin (5-HT) and noradrenaline. Until recently it was considered that hypericin was the principal active ingredient in hypericum, since this inhibits monoamine oxidase and interacts with relevant receptors (Raffa, 1998). However, another constituent of the plant, hyperforin, has recently been shown to be even more active, specifically as an inhibitor of the re-uptake of 5-HT, noradrenaline and dopamine (Chatterjee *et al.*, 1998). Interestingly, the crude plant extract also interacts with high affinity at the $GABA_A$ and $GABA_B$ receptors (Cott, 1997), which has raised the question of whether the transmitter GABA is also intimately involved in the disease. It would be remarkable, but not inconsistent with past history, if plant chemicals and their actions provided new insights into disease mechanisms at the present time, when most research is either descriptive (of the disease) or model (e.g. experimental animal) based.

Parkinson's disease

Rectification of the movement disorder in Parkinson's disease is generally achieved using L-dopa, the natural precursor of the transmitter dopamine, which is deficient in the diseased brain. This therapy evolved from the 'rational' approach to disease treatment. First a deficit of dopamine was discovered in the brains of patients affected, and then the logical chemical treatment – using L-dopa as a precursor of dopamine – was tested (familiar to many through the film *The Awakenings*, based on Oliver Sacks' book). However, before this time it was customary to treat patients with anticholinergics such as atropine, originally derived from belladonna or datura, which restored the dopaminergic–cholinergic imbalance by reducing the activity of the latter. Equally interesting is the traditional use in India of the bean *Mucuna pruriens*, which actually contains L-dopa. The alkaloids from the fungus ergot *Claviceps purpurea* have provided the basis of several recently introduced anti-Parkinsonian drugs such as cabergoline and terguride. These compounds are dopamine D2 receptor agonists, which are co-administered with L-dopa. Ergot was traditionally known as a hallucinogen, but also had beneficial properties because of its vasoconstrictive activity which is also associated with the dopaminergic compounds present (utilized in stimulating uterine contraction and preventing excessive bleeding at childbirth). This is a good example of how knowing the pharmacological basis underlying one traditional use may provide applications in other therapeutic areas. The remarkable success of empirical remedies such as these, which it transpires contain the same chemicals and target the same systems as those later 'discovered' scientifically, continues to provide the incentive to investigate ethnopharmacological medicines further.

Anxiolytics and hypnotics

The first modern tranquillizer, reserpine, was extracted from the roots of *Rauvolfia serpentina* in the mid-twentieth century. The use of this herbal material for the treatment of various forms of 'madness' was recorded in ancient Sanskrit texts, and it had been used in India for centuries.

The underground organs of members of the genus *Valeriana* (Valerianaceae) are used in the traditional medicine of many cultures as mild anxiolytics and to aid the induction of sleep. *V. officinalis* is the species most commonly used in northern Europe and it still retains its official pharmacopoeial status, although it is most commonly encountered as an ingredient of herbal medicines. This plant is still the subject of research aimed at establishing the chemical and pharmacological basis of the activity, which has been clearly shown in a number of animal and clinical studies (Houghton, 1997). The constituents of the volatile oil are very variable due to population differences in genetics, and to environmental factors. The major constituents include the monoterpene, bornyl acetate, and the sesquiterpene, valerenic acid, which is characteristic of the species, in addition to other types of sesquiterpene. Some of these have been shown to have a direct action on the amygdaloid nucleus of the brain, an area concerned with emotional response, and valerenic acid has been shown to inhibit enzyme-induced breakdown of GABA in the brain, resulting in sedation. The non-volatile monoterpenes known as valepotriates were first isolated in 1966 (Inouye, 1991), and contribute to the overall activity by possessing sedative activity based on the CNS, although the mode of action is not yet clear. The valepotriates themselves act as prodrugs and are transformed into homobaldrinal, which has been shown to reduce spontaneous mobility in mice. More recent studies have shown that aqueous extracts of the roots contain appreciable amounts of GABA, which could directly cause sedation, although there is some controversy surrounding the bioavailability of this compound. Another recent finding is the presence of a lignan, hydroxypinoresinol, and its ability to bind to benzodiazepine receptors (Houghton, 1997).

Future prospects

Herbal texts such as those cited in the section on Alzheimer's disease contain innumerable references to other plants used to treat disorders of the CNS. A few examples include the anxiolytic or sedative effects of vervain (*Verbena officinalis*) and chamomile (*Chamaemelum nobile*), the stimulant effects of mint (*Mentha*) species and the antidepressant effects of borage (*Borago officinalis*), mugwort (*Artemisia vulgaris*) and balm. It would be surprising if amongst these plant applications there are not still many new discoveries to be made, in the context of relevant scientific models. Medical herbalists in the West have continued the traditions of plant medicine, and to them such plant applications are standard. However, to convince practitioners of orthodox medicine, clinical trial-based evidence of the safety and efficacy of plant extracts or chemicals is essential. In some respects the issue of safety is already established through centuries of experience, provided attention is paid to identifying precisely the plant species, parts to be used, and recommended methods of extraction and dosage. It might even be suggested that the medicinal use of an indigenous plant by a human society across millennia could have led, in earlier days of survival selection, to individuals less vulnerable to adverse effects and more able to profit from the beneficial effects. This, together with the phenomena of synergy and polypharmacy, provides an appeal of plant medicine that is likely to flourish in the next millennium. The issue of how future phytotherapeutic research should be funded to support definitive clinical trials and relevant basic research is unresolved, with many companies that market plant products lacking the major research resources of the pharmaceutical industry, and the latter generally depending on novel synthetic chemicals or analogues for commercial viability.

The archival discovery, clinical trials conducted in the absence of pre-clinical drug development and current prescription of the new anti-malarial artemesin derived from one of the wormwood species (*Artemisia annua*) does, however, establish an important precedent for the integration of phytotherapy into evidence-based clinical practice.

Acknowledgements

Sections of this article are based on a previous publication in the *Journal of Alternative and Complementary Medicine* (Perry *et al.*, 1998). Lesley Milner very kindly provided the information on medieval medical practices, and many thanks are due to Dawn Houghton for secretarial assistance.

References

Bartram, T. (1995). *Encyclopaedia of Herbal Medicine*. Grace Publishers.

Bhattacharya, S. K. and Kumar, A. (1997). Effect of Trasina, an Ayurvedic herbal formulation, on experimental models of Alzheimer's disease and central cholinergic markers in rats. *J. Alt. Complem. Med.*, **3**, 327–336.

Bhattacharya, S. K., Kumar, A. and Jaiswal, A. K. (1995). Effect of Mentat[®], a herbal formulation, on experimental models of Alzheimer's disease and central cholinergic markers in rats. *Fitoterapia*, **66**, 216–222.

Bruno, C., Cuppini, R., Sartini, S. *et al.* (1993). Regeneration of motor nerves in bilobalide-treated rats. *Planta Medica*, **59**, 302–7.

Burkard, G. and Lehri, S. (1991). Verhältnis von demenzen vom multi-infarkt und vom Alzheimertyp in ärzlichen praxen. Diagnostiche und Therapeutische Konsequenzen am beispiel eines Ginkgo-biloba-präparates. *Münch. Med. Wschr.*, **133** (Suppl. 1), 38–43.

Chatterjee, S. S., Bhattacharya, S. K., Wonnemann, M. *et al.* (1998). Hyperforin as a possible antidepressant component of hypericum extracts. *Life Sci.*, **63**(6), 499–510.

Cheng, D. H. and Tang, X. C. (1998). Comparative studies of huperzine A, E2020 and tacrine on behavioural and cholinesterase activities.

Pharmacol. Biochem. Behav., **60**, 377–86.

Cheng, D. H., Ren, H. and Tang, X. C. (1996). Huperzine A: a novel promising acetylcholinesterase inhibitor. *NeuroReport*, **8**, 97–101.

Clementi, F., Court, J. A. and Perry, E. K. (1999). Neuronal nicotinic receptor involvement in disease. In *Handbook of Experimental Pharmacology* (F. Clementi *et al.*, eds), in press.

Coghan, T. (1584) *The Haven of Health*.

Cott, J. M. (1997). In vitro receptor binding and enzyme inhibition by *Hypericum perforatum* extract. *Pharmacopsychiatry*, **30**(2), 108–12.

Court, J. A. and Perry, E. K. (1994). CNS nicotine receptors: therapeutic target in neurodegeneration. *CNS Drugs*, **2**, 216–33.

Court, J., Lloyd, S., Piggott, M. *et al.* (1998). Effect of tobacco on nicotinic receptor in human brain. *Neuroscience.* **87**, 63–70.

Culpeper, N. (1652). *Culpeper's Complete Herbal* (facsimile of original 1652 publication). Foulsham & Co.

Evelyn, J. (1699). *Acetaria* (cited in Le Strange, 1977).

Everard, G. (1659). *Panacea or the Universal Medicine*.

Fu, F. Z. and Fruehof, H. (1995). Senile dementia and Alzheimer's disease, 1995. Collection of unedited papers from a review of Chinese Language Literature produced for the Institute of Tradition Medicine, Portland Oregon (http//www.europa.com/˜itm/alzheim.htm).

Fulton, B. and Benfield, P. (1996). Galanthamine. *Drugs Aging*, **9**, 60–65.

Gerard, J. (1597). *The Herball, or General Historie of Plantes*, London.

Grieve, M. (1931) *A Modern Herbal*. Jonathan Cape, reprinted by Penguin Books Ltd, 1980.

Halpert, B. P. (1983). Development of the term 'senility' as a medical diagnosis. *Minn. Med.*, **66**, 421–4.

Hann, R. M., Pagan, O. R., Gregory, L. *et al.* (1998). Characterization of cembranoid interaction with the nicotinic acetylcholine receptor. *J. Pharmacol. Exp. Therapeut.*, **287**, 253–60.

Hill, J. (1755). *The Family Herbal*.

Hirokawa, S., Nose, M., Ishige, A. *et al.* (1996). Effect of Hachimi-jio-gan on scopolamine-induced memory impairment and on acetylcholine content in rat brain. *J. Ethnopharmacol.*, **50**, 77–84.

Houghton, P. J. (ed.) (1997). *Valerian*. Harwood.

Houghton, P. J. (1999). Roots of remedies: plants, people and pharmaceuticals. *Chem. Indust.*, January, 15–19.

Hughes, J., Smith, T. W., Kasterlitz, H. W. *et al.* (1975). Identification of two related pentapeptides from the brain with potent opiate agonist activists. *Nature*, **258**, 577–595.

Hunt, T. (1990). *Popular Medicine in Thirteenth Century England*. D. S. Brewer.

Hwang, S. Y., Chang, Y. P., Byun, S. J. *et al.* (1996). An acetylcholinesterase inhibitor isolated from corydalis tuber and its mode of action. *Kor. J. Pharmacog.*, **27**, 91–5.

Inouye, H. (1991). Iridoids pp. 99–144. In *Methods of Plant Biochemistry*, Vol. 7 Terpenoids. (Eds: Charlwood, B. V., Banthorpe, D. V.) Academic Press.

Kanowski, S., Herrmann, W. M., Stephan, K. *et al.* (1996). Proof of efficacy of the *Ginkgo biloba* special extract EGb 761 in outpatients suffering from mild to moderate primary degenerative dementia of the Alzheimer type or multi-infarct dementia. *Pharmacopsychiatry,* **29**, 47–56.

Karch, S. B. (1997). *A Brief History of Cocaine.* CRC Press, Boca Raton.

Kleijnen, J. and Knipschild, P. (1992). *Ginkgo biloba* for cerebral insufficiency. *Br. J. Clin. Pharmacol.,* **34**, 352–8.

Le Bars, P. L., Katz, M. M., Berman, N. *et al.* (1997). A placebo-controlled, double-blind randomized trial of an extract *Ginkgo biloba* for dementia. *JAMA,* **278**, 1327–32.

Lee, P. N. (1994). Smoking and Alzheimer's disease: a review of the epidemiological evidence. *Neuroepidemiology,* **13**, 131–44.

Le Strange, R. (1977). *A History of Herbal Plants.* Morrison & Gibb.

Lewis, R., Wake, G., Court, G. *et al.* (1999). Non-ginsenoside nicotinic activity in ginseng species. *Phytother. Res.,* **13**, 59–64.

Lim, J. H., Wen, T. C., Matsuda, S. *et al.* (1997). Protection of ischaemic hippocampal neurons by ginsenoside RBI, a main ingredient of ginseng root. *Neurosci. Res.,* **28**, 191–200.

Linde, K., Ramirez, G., Mulrow, C. D. *et al.* (1996). St John's wort for depression – an overview and meta-analysis of randomised clinical trials. *Br. Med. J.,* **313**(7052), 253–8.

London Dispensary (1696) cited by Grieve, 1931.

Mahendra, B. (1987). *Dementia: A Survey of the Syndrome of Dementia.* MTP Press.

Mann, J. (1992). *Murder, Magic and Medicine.* Oxford University Press.

Manyam, B. (1999). Dementia in Ayurveda. *J. Compl. Alt. Med.,* **5**, 61–88.

Matthee, R. (1995). Exotic substances: the introduction and global spread of tobacco, coffee, cocoa, tea and distilled liquor, 16th to 18th centuries. In *Drugs and Narcotics in History* (R. Porter and M. Teich, eds) pp. 24–51. Cambridge University Press.

McIntyre, A. (1996). *The Complete Floral Healer.* Gaia Books Ltd.

Mills, S. Y. (1993). *The Essential Book of Herbal Medicine.* Penguin Books.

Mitchell, S. (1993). Aromatherapy's effectiveness in disorders associated with dementia. *Int. J. Aromather.,* **5**, 20–23.

Miyazawa, M., Watanabe, H. and Kameoka, H. (1997). Inhibition of acetylcholinesterase activity by monoterpenoids with a p-methane skeleton. *J. Agric. Food Chem.,* **45**, 677–9.

Nitta, H., Matsumoto, K., Shimiza, M. *et al.* (1995). Panax ginseng extract improves the scopolamine-induced disruption of 8-arm radial maze performance in rats. *Pharmaceut. Bull.,* **18**, 1439.

Ohta, H., Ni, J. W., Matsumoto, K. *et al.* (1993). Paeony and its major constituent, paeoniflorin, improve radial maze performance impaired by scopolamine in rats. *Pharmacol. Biochem. Behav.,* **45**, 719–23.

Park, C. H., Kim, S. H., Choi, W. *et al.* (1996). A novel anticholinesterase and antiamnesic activities of dehydroevodiamie, a constituent of *Evodia rutaecarpa. Planta Medica,* **62**, 405–9.

Pereira, E. F., Reinhadt-Maelicke, S., Schrattenholz, A. *et al.* (1993). Identification and functional characterization of a new agonist site on nicotinic acetylcholine receptors of cultured hippocampal neurones. *J. Pharmacol. Exp. Ther.*, **265**, 1474–91.

Perry, E. K. (1997). Cholinergic phytochemicals: from magic to medicine. *Aging Mental Health*, **1**, 23–32.

Perry, E. K. and Perry, R. H. (1995). Acetylcholine and hallucinations: disease-related compared to drug-induced alterations in human consciousness. *Brain Cogn.*, **28**, 240–58.

Perry, E. K., Pickering, A. T., Wang, W. W. *et al.* (1998). Medicinal plants and Alzheimer's disease: integrating ethnobotanical and contemporary scientific evidence. *J. Alt. Compl. Med.*, **4**, 419–28.

Perry, N., Court, G., Bidet. N. *et al.* (1996). European herbs with cholinergic activities: potential in dementia therapy. *Int. J. Geriatr. Psychiatr.*, **11**, 1063–9.

Perry, N. S. L., Houghton, P. J., Jenner, P. and Perry, E. K. (1999a). *In vitro* inhibition of human erythrocyte acetylcholinesterase by *Salvia lavandulaefolia* essential oil and its constituents (in press).

Perry, N., Howes, M.-J., Houghton, P. J. and Perry, E. (1999b). Why sage may be a wise remedy: effects of salvia on the nervous system. In *Salvia* (S. Kintzias, ed). Harwood.

Pert, C. B. and Snyder, S. H. (1973). Opiate receptor: demonstration in nervous tissue. *Science*, **179**, 1011–1014.

Price, S. and Price, L. (1995). *Aromatherapy for Health Professionals*. Churchill Livingstone.

Raffa, R. B. (1998). Screen of receptor and uptake-site activity of hypericin component of St John's wort reveals sigma receptor binding. *Life Sci.*, **62**(16), 265–70.

Reid, D. P. (1986). *Chinese Herbal Medicine*. Shambala Publications.

Riddle, J. M. (1985). *Dioscorides on Pharmacy and Medicine*. University of Texas Press.

Salim, K. N., McEwan, B. S. and Chao, H. M. (1997). Ginsenoside Rb1 regulates ChAT, NGF and trkA mRNA expression in the rat brain. *Mol. Brain Res.*, **47**, 177–182.

Schliebs, R., Liebmann, A., Bhattacharya, S. K. *et al.* (1997). Systemic administration of defined extracts of *Withania somnifera* (Indian ginseng) and Shilajit differentially affects cholinergic but not glutamatergic and GABAergic markers in rat brain. *Neurochem. Int.*, **30**, 181–90.

Schultes, R. E. (1993). Plants in treating senile dementia in the Northwest Amazon. *J. Ethnopharmacol.*, **38**, 129–35.

Schultes, R. E. and Hofmann, A. (1992). *Plants of the Gods*. Healing Arts Press.

Skolnick, A. A. (1997). Old Chinese herbal medicine used for fever yields possible new Alzheimer disease therapy. *JAMA*, **277**, 776.

Smith, P. F., MacLennan, K. and Darlington, C. L. (1996). The neuroprotective properties of the *Ginkgo biloba* leaf: A review of the possible relationship to platelet-activating factor. *J. Ethnopharmacol.*, **56**, 131–9.

Taylor, J. E. (1986). Neuromediator binding to receptors in the rat brain. The effect of chronic administration of *Ginkgo biloba* extract. *Presse*

Medicale-Paris, **15**, 1491–3.

Ulrich, Y., Johannson-Locher, G., Seiler, W. D. and Stahelin, H. B. (1997). Does smoking protect from Alzheimer's disease? Alzheimer-type changes in 301 unselected brains from patients with known smoking history. *Acta Neuropathol.,* **94**, 450–54.

Vesper, J. and Hadgen, K. D. (1994). Efficacy of *Ginkgo biloba* in 90 outpatients with cerebral insufficiency caused by old age. *Phytomedicine,* **1**, 9–16.

Wake, G., Court, J., Pickering, A. *et al.* (1999). Nicotinic receptor activity in European plants with a tradition of memory improvement. *J. Ethnopharmacol.,* in press.

Watanabe, H., Ni, J. W., Ohta, H. *et al.* (1991). A Kampo prescription, Shimotsu-to, improves scopolamine-induced spatial cognitive deficits in rats. *Jpn. J. Psychopharmacol.,* **11**, 215–22.

Wen, T. C., Yoshimura, H., Matsuda, S. *et al.* (1996). Ginseng root prevents learning disability and neuronal loss in gerbils with 5-minute forebrain ischemia. *Acta Neuropathol.,* **91**, 15–22.

Wren, R. C. (1985). *Potter's New Cyclopaedia of Botanical Drugs and Preparations.* The C. W. Daniel Co. Ltd.

Xu, S. S., Gao, Z. X., Weng, Z. *et al.* (1995). Efficacy of tablet huperzine-A on memory, cognition and behaviour in Alzheimer's disease. *Chung-Kuo Yao Li Hsueh Pao-Acta Pharmacologica Sinica,* **16**, 391–5.

2

Phytotherapy: consumer and pharmacist perspectives

J. Barnes

Introduction

It is widely accepted that there is an increasing use of herbal remedies (also known as phytomedicines) by the general public to replace or complement conventional medicines (Newall *et al.*, 1996). This resurgence of interest in herbal remedies is largely consumer-driven, and comes alongside the public's increasing interest and confidence in self-medication (Blenkinsopp and Bradley, 1996). Pharmacies have become one of the main distribution channels for herbal products, and the pharmacist is the healthcare professional who is most accessible to users of herbal remedies.

This chapter will explore in more depth some of the perspectives of the consumer and the pharmacist with regard to herbal medicines. It is written largely, although not entirely, from a UK viewpoint.

Increasing use of herbal medicine and herbal medicine practitioners

UK and rest of Europe

There have been several analyses of the herbal medicines markets of different countries.

A report by the Mintel market research group on retail sales of complementary medicines (defined in its study as licensed herbal medicines, homoeopathic remedies and essential oils) showed that licensed herbals make up more than 50 per cent of the total complementary medicines market in the UK (Mintel International Group, 1997). Retail sales of herbal products were estimated to be worth £38 million in 1996, compared with £27.2 million in 1991; however, £38 million is likely to be a gross underestimate since Mintel excluded garlic, ginkgo and unlicensed herbal products from its analysis. Since the majority of sales of herbal products in the UK are of unlicensed preparations, the figure for sales of *all* herbal products is likely to be several-fold higher. The use of herbal products is widespread across Europe – the total over-the-counter (OTC) market for herbal remedies in 1991 was said to be worth £1.45 billion (Fisher and Ward, 1994). Blumenthal *et al.* (1998) cite an estimate of US$7000 million for 1996 retail sales of herbal remedies in the European Union.

A detailed analysis of the herbal medicines market in Europe comes from the Institute of Medical Statistics (IMS) Self-Medication International, which published its *Herbals in Europe* report in 1998 (IMS, 1998). The IMS analysis used the European Scientific Co-operative on Phytotherapy (ESCOP) definition for herbal medicinal products and included branded products only. Sales values were calculated at ex-manufacturer prices, i.e. the price at which the manufacturer sells to the wholesaler, and given in US dollars. According to the report, Germany and France make up more than 70 per cent of the European market.

In Germany, total sales of herbal products were US$1.8 billion in 1997, making up a third of the total market for OTC products. Pharmacies represented 84 per cent of sales, with drug stores (11 per cent) and supermarkets (5 per cent) making up the remainder. The leading categories of herbal products in Germany were cough/cold and circulatory products. Growth in the German herbals market, however, halted in 1997, mainly as a result of pressure from the German sick funds (IMS, 1998). In France, where figures currently comprise pharmacy sales only, total sales of herbal products reached US$1.1 billion in 1997, representing 28 per cent of the total OTC market. Here, herbal circulatory products was a leading category (IMS, 1998).

Although self-medication accounts for the vast majority of herbal remedy use, in the UK at least, some individuals do of course consult medical herbalists. A Gallup poll in 1986 reported that 2 per cent of the sample surveyed ($n = 1045$) had at some point consulted a herbalist and that 3 per cent knew of a family member who had done so (Gallup, 1986). In 1995, the Consumers' Association in the UK carried out a survey of 20 000 individuals to determine the level of use of complementary medicine (Consumers' Association, 1995). Of the 44 per cent who replied ($n = 8745$), 31 per cent had consulted a practitioner of complementary medicine at some time, and of these 6 per cent ($n = 163$) had consulted a herbalist in the previous 12 months. It is not easy to obtain a clear picture of the use of medical herbalists from these figures; however, if it is assumed that all other individuals surveyed had not consulted a medical herbalist in the previous 12 months, then the 163 individuals who had done so represent less than 1 per cent of the total sample.

United States

Brevoort has provided detailed overviews of the US market for herbal remedies (Brevoort, 1996, 1998). In 1994, annual retail sales of botanical medicines were estimated to be around US$1.6 billion; in 1998, the figure was closer to US$4 billion (Brevoort, 1998).

Some of the best data regarding trends in the use of complementary therapies come from Eisenberg and colleagues, who conducted two telephone surveys of US adults using random digit dialling (Eisenberg *et al.*, 1993, 1998). The surveys were carried out in 1991 (to determine patterns of use during 1990) and 1997–1998 (to determine patterns of use during 1997), and involved over 1500 and over 2000 individuals respectively. Herbal medicine was one of the therapies showing the greatest increase over this time period – there was a statistically significant increase in unsupervised use (i.e. self-medication) of herbal medicine from 2.5 per cent of the sample in 1990 to 12.5 per cent in 1997 (Eisenberg *et al.*, 1998). The proportion of US adults who had visited a practitioner of herbal medicine in the 12 months preceding the survey had also markedly increased, from around 10.2 per cent in 1990 to 15.1 per cent in 1997. Interestingly, the mean number of visits to a herbal practitioner per user had decreased over this time period, from 8.1 in 1990 to 2.9 in 1997. Extrapolation of figures from the 1997 survey (Eisenberg *et al.*, 1998) for self-reported expenditure on herbal products to the whole of the US population provided an estimate of over US$5 billion (the 1990 survey did not include questions on expenditure on herbal products).

Eisenberg and colleagues pointed out some limitations to their studies: the surveys were restricted to English speakers with telephones; they relied on self-reported herbal product use; the response rates were 60 and 67 per cent for 1997 and 1990 respectively and it is possible that this may have led to an overestimation of use of complementary therapies; and financial incentives were used in 1997 but not 1990 and it is not known whether this may have introduced any bias (Eisenberg *et al.*, 1998).

Why do people use herbal remedies and for which conditions?

Reasons for use of herbal remedies

Reasons for the increasing use of herbal remedies are many and complex, but are likely to include the following:

- Increasing consumer interest and confidence in self-medication
- The belief that herbal remedies are natural and safe
- Concern about the adverse effects of conventional drugs
- Disappointment with the effectiveness of conventional medicine, particularly in chronic conditions
- The desire for a more natural lifestyle.

Important work in this area has been carried out by Furnham (1997), although his group's work concentrated on patients' use of practitioners rather than self-treatment and did not focus specifically on herbal medicine. In summary, Furnham reported that it appears that the use of complementary medicine is not because of an outright rejection of conventional medicine, but more to do with users' belief that they are in control of their own health. It also appears that people may consult different practitioners for different reasons.

Astin has also carried out a study investigating why people use alternative medicine (Astin, 1998). He reported that users of alternative medicine were not so doing because of a dissatisfaction with conventional medicine, but because they found alternative medicine to be more congruent with their own values, beliefs and philosophical orientations toward health and life.

Conditions treated

Eisenberg and colleagues found that of the most frequently reported medical conditions in their 1997 survey, allergies, insomnia, 'lung problems' and digestive problems were the conditions for which herbal remedies were among the therapies most commonly used (Eisenberg *et al.*, 1998).

Several studies and review papers have focused on the use of complementary therapies by certain patient groups, such as those with asthma (Lamb and Cantrill, 1995; Ernst, 1998a), cancer (Ernst and Cassileth, 1998), depression (Ernst *et al.*, 1998) and rheumatological conditions (Ernst, 1998b), and report varying levels of use of herbal medicine by these types of patients. Herbal remedies are not only used by adults – again, studies and reviews have investigated the use of herbal (and other complementary remedies) in children (for example, Ernst, 1999).

Users of herbal remedies: characteristics, behaviour and perceptions

Barnes and colleagues conducted a survey of users of herbal

remedies, mainly to explore if there is any user bias in how suspected adverse reactions to herbal remedies and conventional OTC medicines might be reported, but also to determine how consumers choose herbal products, where they purchase them and their use of other non-prescription products (Barnes *et al.*, 1998).

Face-to-face interviews with herbal remedy users were carried out using a structured questionnaire in six Boots pharmacies and six Holland & Barrett healthfood stores in England and Wales. The remainder of this subsection discusses mainly data from this study.

Characteristics of herbal remedy users

Of 690 individuals who agreed to be interviewed, 175 (25.4 per cent) stated that they did not use herbal remedies and thus these interviews were terminated. In total, 515 users of herbal remedies were interviewed. Eighty-two per cent of respondents were female; the ethnic origin of respondents was predominantly Caucasian (91 per cent). The age distribution of respondents was as follows: less than 20 years, 2 per cent; 20–29 years, 15 per cent; 30–39 years, 20 per cent; 40–49 years, 24 per cent; 50–59 years, 19 per cent; more than 60 years, 20 per cent.

Behaviour of herbal remedy users

Of the respondents, 62 per cent said they were 'regular' users of herbal remedies and 38 per cent 'occasional' users, although these terms were not defined so the breakdown is tentative. Respondents were asked to name up to three herbal remedies that they used most commonly. Evening primrose oil/starflower oil (23 per cent), garlic (27 per cent) and herbal sleep/sedatives (25 per cent) accounted for 75 per cent of all products named ($n = 687$) (unpublished observations). Another survey involving 136 customers (70.1 per cent response rate) who had purchased dietary supplements in either of two US healthfood stores reported that, of the 805 supplements named by respondents, 84.3 per cent were taken for disease prevention and 'wellness', with the remainder being taken to treat perceived health problems (Eliason *et al.*, 1997). Herbal products, including garlic and ginseng (grouped separately by the authors of the study), accounted for 27 per cent of all named products; garlic, ginseng and *Ginkgo biloba* were the herbal products most commonly named.

Barnes and colleagues reported that 78 per cent of herbal remedy users in their survey also used vitamins/minerals or food supplements, 49 per cent used complementary remedies other than herbals, and 81 per cent were also users of conventional OTC medicines (these figures do not necessarily reflect concurrent use) (Barnes *et al.*, 1998). Based on figures from their 1997 survey, Eisenberg and colleagues estimated that 15 million adults in the US who are regularly taking prescription medicines are concurrently using at least one herbal and/or high-dose vitamin preparation (i.e. 18 per cent of all prescription medicine users) (Eisenberg *et al.*, 1998). Furthermore, the disclosure rate to physicians of complementary therapy use was less than 40 per cent in both the 1990 and 1997 surveys. Similarly, Eliason *et al.* (1997) reported that of the 805 dietary supplements named by respondents, 85.3 per cent were taken for a benefit for which users had not consulted their physician.

Barnes *et al.* (1998) reported that 6 per cent of respondents in their survey chose herbal remedies on the basis of a doctor's, pharmacist's, or herbal practitioner's recommendation alone – that is, where there is some informed and/or professional advice available. By contrast, 83 per cent chose only on the basis of one or more of the following: other complementary-medicine practitioner's recommendation; own knowledge; friend or family member's recommendation; media advertising; by browsing in shops; other basis. The remaining 11 per cent chose on the basis of information from both sources. A similar observation was made by Eliason *et al.* (1997) who reported that, of the 805 dietary supplements named by respondents, 79 per cent were taken on the basis of the users' own information or investigation (e.g. books, magazines, 'word of mouth'), 8.7 per cent on the recommendation of a nutritionist, 6.1 per cent on a physician's recommendation and 5.8 per cent on another healthcare professional's recommendation.

In addition to purchasing herbal remedies from pharmacies (64 per cent) and healthfood stores (54 per cent), the types of outlet in which their survey was conducted, Barnes *et al.* (1998) found that some respondents also claimed to obtain herbal remedies from supermarkets/grocery stores (10 per cent), by mail order (5 per cent), from the garden or countryside (1 per cent), or from some other source (6 per cent) (data not mutually exclusive).

Perceptions of herbal remedy users

It has been reported that following a 'serious side effect' (defined as a symptom that was 'worrying or alarming'), 156 respondents (30.3 per cent) would consult their GP irrespective of whether an adverse drug reaction (ADR) was associated with the use of a herbal remedy or a conventional OTC medicine, and that 221 respondents

(42.9 per cent) would not consult their GP for a serious side effect associated with either type of preparation (Barnes *et al.*, 1998). One hundred and thirty-four respondents (26.0 per cent) would consult their GP for a serious ADR to a conventional OTC medicine but not for a similar ADR to a herbal remedy, whereas four respondents (0.8 per cent) would consult their GP for a serious ADR to a herbal remedy but not for a similar ADR to a conventional OTC medicine. Thus, there appears to be a marked proportion of herbal remedy users who would act differently for a serious side effect depending on whether it was associated with a herbal remedy or a conventional OTC medicine.

There may be several reasons for this – herbal remedies are used largely on a self-treatment basis in the UK, and users may not realize that they can consult their GP about such products or may be reluctant to admit herbal product use, particularly if they experience an adverse event. Barnes *et al.* (1998) also appear to have uncovered a possible under-utilization of the pharmacist by herbal remedy consumers for advice on adverse effects – overall, only 15 per cent of respondents said they would consult a pharmacist for an adverse effect to a conventional OTC medicine and/or a herbal remedy.

There are some limitations to these findings: herbal remedy consumers were asked a hypothetical question and it is possible that they may act differently if they experienced an actual adverse event; the definition of a 'serious side effect' was not validated; and it is not known whether the apparent consumer confusion over what is a herbal remedy could have influenced the results. Nevertheless, it does appear that some aspects of consumers' perceived behaviour with regard to reporting adverse effects associated with herbal remedies may have implications for herbal pharmacovigilance (Barnes *et al.*, 1998).

Thirty-one respondents said that they had experienced side effects associated with herbal remedies; however, despite interviewers' use of photographs of common herbal products to assist consumers in identifying herbal remedies, 10 of these reports related to non-herbal complementary remedies such as minerals and homoeopathic remedies, illustrating that there appears to be consumer confusion over what is and what is not a herbal remedy (Barnes *et al.*, 1998). Thus, 21 reports of suspected side effects associated with herbals were reported in the survey. These are perceived adverse effects and, despite attempts to do so, even those cases where consumers claimed to have reported the event to their doctor could not be confirmed. Nevertheless, such reports give some indication of how consumers might act upon experiencing an adverse event that they associate with a herbal remedy; three consumers claimed to have reported the event to their GP, whilst the majority of consumers stopped taking the preparation concerned.

Another survey solicited reports from the public of perceived adverse effects associated with complementary therapies. Twenty-four such reports were received for herbal products although again, despite attempts to do so, even those cases where consumers claimed to have reported the event to their doctor could not be confirmed (Abbot *et al.*, 1998).

The role of the pharmacist in herbal medicine

Since herbal remedies are widely sold in pharmacies, and given that the community pharmacist is the healthcare professional who is most accessible to users of such remedies, it is likely that there is a key role for pharmacists in advising patients and consumers about the safe and effective use of herbal remedies. For example, pharmacists are ideally placed to advise patients about the use of herbal remedies for minor ailments, and on the potential for interactions between herbal remedies and conventional medicines. Furthermore, it has been recognized by the UK Committee on Safety of Medicines (CSM) that pharmacists have a role to play in adverse reaction reporting for herbal remedies. In April 1997, the CSM extended its yellow card scheme for adverse reaction reporting to all hospital pharmacists and, as part of a pilot study, to community pharmacists in the four CSM monitoring regions (CSM, 1997a); community pharmacists were asked to focus on areas of limited reporting by doctors, i.e. over-the-counter medicines and (licensed and unlicensed) herbal products (CSM, 1997b).

However, at present the level of intervention of the pharmacist in decisions on herbal remedy use is almost certainly well below optimal for several reasons. First, the vast majority of herbal remedies on sale in the UK is on the General Sales List, therefore such remedies do not have to be sold under the supervision of a pharmacist and can be sold in retail outlets other than pharmacies. Even consumers purchasing herbal remedies from a pharmacy may not have any contact with a pharmacist, or indeed any other member of pharmacy staff. Where a pharmacist is involved in the sale of a herbal remedy, he or she may not question the consumer about the use of the product; also, pharmacists may not routinely ask patients specifically about their use of herbal remedies when giving advice on conventional medicines, nor have the facility to record such use on patient medication records. In any case, some patients and consumers may have little knowledge of the herbal products they are using;

some may even be reluctant to admit to herbal product use.

A key factor in pharmacists' reluctance to question patients and consumers about their use of herbal remedies may be that pharmacists feel that their knowledge of such remedies is inadequate. There has been a decline in pharmacognosy in UK schools of pharmacy over the years, to the point where few schools now have units strong in pharmacognosy education and research. Although some schools of pharmacy do provide undergraduate training in aspects of complementary remedies, the general lack of teaching in pharmacognosy has contributed to pharmacists' lack of knowledge about herbal remedies (Houghton, 1997).

Phillipson (1999) has emphasized the need for a renewed emphasis on pharmacognosy in UK schools of pharmacy, and there have been other calls for both undergraduate teaching and continuing education for pharmacists in herbal and other complementary remedies and therapies (Launso, 1995; Abdel-Rahman and Nahata, 1997). While there are now several sources of reliable information on herbal medicine available for pharmacists and other healthcare professionals (for example, HMSO, 1995; Newall *et al.*, 1996; Tyler, 1996; Barnes, 1998; Schulz *et al.*, 1998; Williamson and Wyandt, 1998), it is likely that more training is required. If pharmacists do not develop research-based knowledge in herbal medicine, there may be implications for pharmaceutical care, and it is possible that other professions will move to meet patients' and consumers' needs (Launso, 1995). If the latter occurs, the resulting situation may not be what is best for the patient or consumer. For example, in a study of advice given by healthfood shop staff to a female researcher posing as a customer with symptoms associated with serious pathology, all but two of the 29 stores recommended a specific therapeutic intervention, whereas only seven of 29 suggested that the 'consumer' should consult her GP (Vickers *et al.*, 1998).

Increasing sales of herbal remedies in pharmacies

Nevertheless, pharmacies have become one of the main distribution channels for herbal products in the UK. The Mintel study reported that 50 per cent of retail sales of herbal products are made from pharmacies, although this may be an overestimate given the bias to licensed herbals only (Mintel International Group, 1997). In April 1997, Brown conducted a survey of a random sample of 400 community pharmacists in Texas, USA. Of the 142 respondents (36.3 per cent response rate), 68.3 per cent reported that herbal products were stocked in the pharmacy in which they practised.

Furthermore, in February 1998 Barnes (Barnes and Abbot, 1999) carried out a cross-sectional survey of 1337 community pharmacists in six regions of the UK (Devon, Cornwall, Manchester, Leeds, Stockport and Bradford). Of the 818 respondents (eligible response rate = 67 per cent), 99 per cent of pharmacies in which respondent pharmacists practised sold at least one type of complementary remedy, including vitamins and minerals. Of these, 76.3 per cent sold herbal remedies, 33.2 per cent sold anthroposophical remedies, and 73.2 per cent sold essential oils (data not mutually exclusive).

Pharmacists' attitudes and perceptions towards herbal medicine

Nelson *et al.* (1990) conducted a survey of US (*n* = 1000) and British (*n* = 750) hospital and community pharmacists to determine pharmacists' knowledge and attitudes towards 'alternative health approaches', including herbal medicine. Response rates were 19.7 per cent and 63.0 per cent for US and British pharmacists respectively. Of the British respondents, 74.4 per cent claimed to 'know something about' or 'know a lot about' herbal remedies, whereas 25.6 per cent perceived that they had 'never heard of' or 'only heard of' such remedies. Figures for US pharmacists were 53.3 per cent and 46.7 per cent for 'know something/a lot about' and 'never/only heard of', respectively. Also, 65 per cent of British pharmacists perceived herbal remedies as 'useful', 7.4 per cent considered them 'useless', and 27.6 per cent did not know how they perceived the usefulness of such remedies. Corresponding figures for US pharmacists were: 'useful', 42.6 per cent; 'useless', 19.8 per cent; and 'don't know', 37.6 per cent.

These differences, which suggest that (at the time of the survey) herbal medicine was more favoured by British than by US pharmacists, were among the largest for all 21 alternative health approaches included in the survey. According to the authors, these differences between British and US pharmacists persisted when the data were analysed according to whether pharmacists worked in community or hospital (Nelson *et al.*, 1990). Proportions of respondents claiming to refer patients to herbal medicine were 4.8 and 7.1 per cent for British and US pharmacists respectively; 6.0 and 7.6 per cent of British and US respectively claimed to have used herbal remedies themselves (differences were statistically non-significant).

There are some limitations to this study: US pharmacists were selected from one region only (Detroit, Michigan) and the response rate from the sample was particularly low; the sampling strategy for British pharmacists is not entirely clear; and there does not appear to have been a follow-up mailing to non-responders from either sample.

Pharmacists' experiences with herbal and other complementary remedies/therapies

Brown (1998) aimed to assess pharmacists' experiences with the use of 'alternative therapies', including herbal remedies, by patients with chronic illnesses. On the basis of pharmacists' experiences with the last 10 patients with chronic disease seen in their pharmacy, it was estimated that 17 per cent of such patients were using some type of alternative therapy for a chronic condition and that 25 per cent had asked pharmacists for information regarding an alternative therapy that they were considering using for treatment of such a condition.

With regard to known users of alternative therapies, pharmacists reported that 25.9 per cent were generally non-compliant with prescribed medication regimens and that 34.3 per cent periodically substituted alternative therapies for prescribed medication. In only 11.1 per cent of the cases had pharmacists documented patients' use of alternative therapies in these patients' pharmacy records, possibly because pharmacy systems are not currently designed to provide this facility. Interestingly, pharmacists practising in pharmacies that stocked herbal products responded to significantly more requests about alternative therapies than pharmacists practising in pharmacies that did not stock such products ($p = 0.02$).

The findings of this survey are limited by the low response rate and the fact that the sample was limited to pharmacists in one state (Texas). The findings, therefore, cannot necessarily be generalized to pharmacists in other states. Also, as far as this chapter is concerned, the survey focused on pharmacists' experiences with patients using 'alternative therapies' in general, and did not ask pharmacists specifically about their experiences of patients using herbal remedies. Nevertheless, the study does show that pharmacists are experiencing a demand for information on alternative therapies and implies that pharmacists should routinely ask patients about their use of such therapies in order to be able to make informed decisions on patient care.

Barnes (Barnes and Abbot, 1999) asked pharmacists if, in the 12 months prior to the survey, they had been asked for complementary remedies specifically by name, and if they had 'recommended' any such remedies when responding to symptoms. Eighty-one per cent of pharmacists said they had been asked for complementary remedies specifically by name, and 58 per cent had 'recommended' complementary remedies. In both cases, herbal remedies represented the greatest proportion of products named (pharmacists were asked to name up to three complementary remedies); 35.2 per cent of all complementary remedies named by pharmacists as being frequently requested by patients/customers, and 35.7 per cent of all complementary remedies suggested to patients/customers by pharmacists. Herbal sleep/sedative products were the most common category of remedy in both cases.

Barnes (Barnes and Abbot, 1999) found that 70 per cent of pharmacists 'rarely' or 'never' ask patients specifically about complementary remedy use when counter prescribing, or when receiving reports of suspected adverse reactions to conventional medicines. Nevertheless, pharmacists do identify or receive reports from consumers of suspected adverse reactions to complementary remedies. Overall, 90 pharmacists provided 107 such reports, 41 of which were associated with herbal remedies and 21 with essential oils. Pharmacists who had undertaken training in some area of complementary medicine were more likely to have provided a report than those who had not undertaken such training ($p < 0.001$). Of the 41 reports associated with herbal remedies, 70 per cent were reported to pharmacists by patients and 28 per cent were identified by the pharmacist. Where information on concurrent medication was provided, in 62 per cent of cases patients were taking herbal remedies concurrently with conventional medicines (Barnes and Abbot, 1999).

There are limitations to these findings: the survey did not involve a random sample of pharmacists and it is possible that pharmacists in other areas may have different experiences with herbal and other complementary remedies; this was a retrospective survey and there may have been inaccurate recall of detail with regard to reports of suspected adverse reactions – indeed some adverse reactions identified by or reported to pharmacists may not have been recalled at all; and no attempt has been made to assess or classify causality of adverse reaction reports although it is precisely reports of suspected adverse reactions that are requested by the UK Committee on Safety of Medicines' yellow card scheme for ADR reporting.

Advising patients about herbal remedies

Although pharmacists on the whole may lack detailed knowledge about specific herbal remedies, there are some general points of which pharmacists should be aware:

- There is a belief among consumers that herbal remedies are 'natural' and 'safe'; however, this is a misconception – herbal remedies can and do cause adverse effects, some of which may be serious.
- Individuals experiencing adverse effects associated with herbal remedies should inform an appropriate healthcare professional.
- Herbal remedies have the potential to interact with conventional medicines.
- Pharmacists should routinely ask patients/consumers specifically about their use of herbal remedies and, where possible, such use should be recorded.
- There is reliable evidence from randomized controlled trials to support the use of specific herbal remedies for symptom relief in specific conditions. However, more research is needed to establish the efficacy and safety of untested remedies.
- As with all drugs, herbal remedies should not be used during pregnancy and lactation unless the potential benefit outweighs the potential risk.
- Patients wishing to consult a herbal medicine practitioner should choose one who is suitably trained, has adequate indemnity and is registered with a professional body.

Conclusion

In conclusion, there is an increasing use of herbal products and herbal practitioners by the general public for a wide range of conditions. Some aspects of consumers' behaviour and perceived behaviour with regard to the use of herbal remedies give cause for concern, and may have implications for herbal safety, herbal pharmacovigilance and pharmaceutical care.

Given the wide availability of herbal remedies from pharmacies, and the accessibility of the pharmacist to users and potential users of such remedies, there exists an opportunity for pharmacists to play a key role in advising patients and consumers on the safe and effective use of herbal products. As highly trained healthcare professionals with expert knowledge of conventional medicines and, in many cases, access to detailed information on at least prescription medicines taken by individual patients, pharmacists are ideally placed to take on a new role in advising on herbal remedies. However, it is likely that changes in pharmacy practice, greater awareness, and increased vigilance on the part of the pharmacist with regard to herbal products are required, together with a commitment to research-led undergraduate and postgraduate training.

References

Abbot, N. C., Hill, M., Barnes, J. *et al.* (1998). Uncovering suspected adverse effects of complementary and alternative medicine. *Int. J. Risk Safety Med.*, **11**, 99–106.

Abdel-Rahman, S. M. and Nahata, M. C. (1997). Perspectives on alternative medicine. *Ann. Pharmacother.*, **31**(11), 1397–1400.

Astin, J. A. (1998). Why patients use alternative medicine. Results of a national study. *JAMA*, **279**, 1548–53.

Barnes, J. (1998). Herbal medicine. *Pharm. J.*, **260**, 344–8.

Barnes, J., Mills, S. Y., Abbot, N. C. *et al.* (1998). Different standards for reporting ADRs to herbal remedies and conventional OTC medicines: face-to-face interviews with 515 users of herbal remedies. *Br. J. Clin. Pharmacol.*, **45**, 496–500.

Barnes, J. and Abbot, N. C. (1999). Experiences with complementary remedies: a survey of community pharmacists. *Pharm. J.*, **263**, R37.

Blenkinsopp, A. and Bradley, C. (1996). Patients, society and the increase in self medication. *Br. Med. J.*, **312**, 629–32.

Blumenthal, M., Busse, W. R., Goldberg, A. *et al.* (eds) (1998). *The Complete German Commission E monographs.* American Botanical Council.

Brevoort, P. (1996). The US botanical market – an overview. *Herbalgram*, **36**, 49–57.

Brevoort, P. (1998). The booming US botanical market. A new overview. *Herbalgram*, **44**, 33–46.

Brown, C. M. (1998). Use of alternative therapies and their impact on compliance: perceptions of community pharmacists in Texas. *J. Am. Pharm. Ass.*, **38**, 603–8.

Consumers' Association (1995). Healthy choice. *Which?* November, 8–13.

CSM (1997a). Extension of the yellow card scheme to pharmacists. *Curr. Problems Pharmacovigilance*, **23**, 3.

CSM (1997b). Pharmacy ADR reporting now official. *Pharm. J.*, **258**, 582.

Eisenberg, D. M., Kessler, R. C., Foster, C. *et al.* (1993). Unconventional medicine in the United States. Prevalence, costs and patterns of use. *New Engl. J. Med.*, **328**, 246–52.

Eisenberg, D. M., Davis, R. B., Ettner, S. L. *et al.* (1998). Trends in alternative medicine use in the United States, 1990–1997. Results of a follow-up national survey. *JAMA*, **280**(18), 1569–75.

Eliason, B. C., Kruger, J., Mark, D. *et al.* (1997). Dietary supplement users: demographics, product use, and medical system interaction. *J. Am. Board Fam. Pract.*, **10**, 265–71.

Ernst, E. (1998a). Complementary therapies for asthma: what patients use. *J. Asthma*, **35**(8), 667–71.

Ernst, E. (1998b). Usage of complementary therapies in rheumatology: a systematic review. *Clin. Rheumatol.*, **17**, 301–5.

Ernst, E. (1999). Prevalence of complementary/alternative medicine for children: a systematic review. *Eur. J. Pediatr.*, **158**, 7–11.

Ernst, E. and Cassileth, B. (1998). The prevalence of complementary/alternative medicine in cancer. A systematic review. *Cancer*, **83**, 777–82.

Ernst, E., Rand, J. I. and Stevinson, C. (1998). Complementary therapies for depression. An overview. *Arch. Gen. Psychiatry,* **55**, 1026–32.

Fisher, P. and Ward, A. (1994). Complementary medicine in Europe. *Br. Med. J.,* **309**, 107–11.

Furnham, A. (1997). Knowledge, attitudes and beliefs of patients of complementary practitioners. In *Complementary Medicine: A Research Perspective* (C. Vincent and A. Furnham, eds), pp. 97–117. Wiley.

Gallup (1986). Alternative medicine. *Omnibus* report.

HMSO (1995). Herbal medicine. In *Complementary Therapies. Centre for Pharmacy Postgraduate Education.* HMSO.

Houghton, P. (1997). Pharmacognosy in the United Kingdom – 1997. *Pharm. Pharmacol. Lett.,* **7**, 2–3.

IMS (1998). *Herbals in Europe.* Institute of Medical Statistics.

Lamb, C. and Cantrill, J. A. (1995). Asthma patients' usage of over-the-counter medicines and complementary remedies. *Pharm. J.,* **254**, 802–4.

Launso, L. (1995). People choose alternative therapies – the consequences for future pharmacy practice. *J. Soc. Adm. Pharm.,* **12**(1), 43–52.

Mintel International Group (1997). *Complementary Medicines.* Mintel International Group Ltd.

Nelson, M. V., Bailie, G. R. and Areny, H. (1990). Pharmacists' perceptions of alternative health approaches – a comparison between US and British pharmacists. *J. Clin. Pharm. Ther.,* **15**, 141–6.

Newall, C. A., Anderson, L. A. and Phillipson, J. D. (1996). *Herbal Medicines. A Guide for Healthcare Professionals.* The Pharmaceutical Press.

Phillipson, J. D. (1999). Useful drugs from plants – it could be yew. *Phytother. Res.,* **13**, 1–7.

Schulz, V., Hänsel, R. and Tyler, V. E. (1998). *Rational Phytotherapy. A Physician's Guide to Herbal Medicine.* Springer-Verlag.

Tyler, V. E. (1996). What pharmacists should know about herbal remedies. *J. Am. Pharm. Ass.,* **36**, 29–37.

Vickers, A., Rees, R. and Robin, A. (1998). Advice given by health food shops: is it clinically safe? *J. R. Coll. Phys. Lond.,* **32**(5), 426–8.

Williamson, J. S. and Wyandt, C. M. (1998). An herbal update. *Drug Topics,* June, 66–75.

3

New targets in phytopharmacology of plants

H. Wagner

Introduction

The goal of modern phytochemical research is to develop preparations derived from herbal drugs of traditional medicine to meet present-day international standards of quality, safety and efficacy.

To reach this goal the following steps are necessary:

- The isolation and structural elucidation of the major constituents of a herbal drug, which might be responsible for its overall pharmacological activity and efficacy.
- The chemical or biological standardization of a phytopreparation according to National Pharmacopoeias; special monographs worked out, for example, by the German Commission E and Keller (1991), WHO (1991) or ESCOP (European Scientific Cooperative of Phytotherapy) (1993) and described in the guidelines of the IFPMA (International Federation of Pharmaceutical Manufacturers' Association (1997). The IFPMA represents the global research-based pharmaceutical industry, and aims to ensure the same standards of safety, quality and efficacy for new medicines as for established ones and more efficient registration for use worldwide. In addition, a guideline for the fingerprint analysis of mixed preparations containing several raw drugs or extracts has been published by Bauer and Tittel (1996).
- Elucidation of the complete profile of pharmacological effects including the molecular biological mechanisms followed by toxicological studies.
- Controlled clinical studies according to good clinical practice.

Whilst identification of the major active constituents and standardization of a herbal drug or phytopreparation is usually possible today with the help of modern 'high tech' methods, the elucidation of the molecular biological mechanisms underlying the overall pharmacological profile of a herbal drug preparation is still in its infancy. It is, however, essential to obtain more detailed information on this area of phytomedicine, since the functional mechanisms hold the key to rational phytotherapy. Furthermore, questions concerning the correct dosages and indications for phytopreparations are waiting to be answered. This goal can be achieved only by a thorough, new approach in phytopharmacological research.

New screening strategies in phytopharmacology

In order to investigate complex systems such as plant drugs and phytopreparations, which consist of many bioactive compounds, the suggestion of the philosopher Descartes should be followed. He proposed that complex systems that cannot easily be analysed by simple means might be investigated by examining the individual parts of the system. In this way, it is hoped that a rational explanation for the whole will emerge. In other words, more-or-less reductionistic research must be carried out with an awareness, however, that this strategy will never quite explain the entire efficacy of the complete complex of active compounds. The term 'the whole is more than the sum of all its individual parts' is certainly applicable to phytopharmaceuticals.

To follow this approach requires the investigation of extract fractions and single constituents of a herbal drug in various bioassays, comparing the results with those of the herbal raw drug or extract. In contrast to former pharmacological investigations, new targets such as enzymes, receptors, cell cultures and gene domains have to be included. The following examples from the author and his colleagues' research work explain this new strategy.

Target-directed phytopharmacology research

Example 1

In an attempt to explain the cardiotonic activity of hawthorn (*Crataegus oxyacantha*) preparations, verified by numerous clinical studies (Tauchert *et al.*, 1994), it was found that the procyanidines and flavon-C-glycosides appear to be the main constituents responsible for pharmacological activity. In an aorta model, an endothelin-dependent smooth muscle relaxing effect was found, which in turn appears to be caused by a phosphodiesterase-inhibiting effect (Franck *et al.*, 1996). The procyanidins also showed an *in vitro* angiotensin-converting enzyme (ACE) inhibiting effect, which accounts for the further dilating effect on blood vessels with a simultaneous reduction in blood pressure (Wagner *et al.*, 1991). The flavon-glycosides act as antioxidants, inhibitors of cyclo-oxygenase and 5-lipoxygenase, such that additional anti-inflammatory and thrombocyte aggregation inhibitory effects can be expected. These results suggest that, in order to increase the efficacy of hawthorn medication, extracts have to be produced which contain both active classes of compounds in enriched form. It seems a reasonable argument, therefore, to standardize these extracts in both classes of compounds. In this context it is of interest that the alcoholic extracts of two South American Cecropia species (*Cecropia hololeuca* and *C. glaziovii*), as well as the African *Musanga cecropioides* plant, were found to have nearly the same composition of bioactive compounds with the same pharmacological activity and therapeutic application (Franck *et al.*, 1996).

Example 2

Water–alcohol extracts of the root of *Urtica dioica* (stinging-nettle root) have long been used and are still in use for the treatment of benign prostate hyperplasia. Several observational and double-blind studies have assessed its clinical efficacy (Schilcher, 1998). The roots contain a mixture of isolectins (UDA), which possess N-acetyl-glucosamine specificity (Peumanns *et al.*, 1984). By using a ^{125}I-labelled epidermal growth factor receptor preparation, it was possible to show that UDA binds to the EGF-receptor of an epidermal cancer cell line CA 431 in a dose-dependent manner (Wagner *et al.*, 1995). This could result in a competitive inhibition of the epidermal growth factor-induced proliferation. In addition, the polysaccharides isolated from the same root showed immunostimulating and anti-inflammatory activity (Wagner *et al.*, 1994). Since the lectins are also absorbed from the gut after oral administration (Geiger, 1998), it is likely that the well-documented clinical efficacy of Urtica preparations is based on a synergism of antiproliferative and anti-inflammatory effects caused by these two water-soluble classes of compounds.

Example 3

Since the pharmacological role of garlic (*Allium sativum*) in the prevention and treatment of cancer and atherosclerosis has received increasing attention and because thorough investigations into the molecular mechanisms of action of garlic compounds are lacking, allicin and ajoene have been investigated in two new *in vitro* models. The first used an apoptosis-inducing model, whereas the second was performed with the inducible nitric oxide synthase (iNOS) from human macrophages.

In the first experiment, it could be shown that ajoene induced apoptosis in human leukaemic cells but not in peripheral mononuclear blood cells of healthy subjects. Ajoene increased the production of intracellular peroxide in a dose- and time-dependent fashion, which could be partially blocked by pre-incubation of the human leukaemic cells with the antioxidant N-acetyl-cysteine. This result suggests that ajoene might induce apoptosis via the stimulation of peroxide production and activation of nuclear factor κB (Dirsch *et al.*, 1998a). This novel aspect is an important step in elucidating the underlying molecular mechanisms of its antitumour action.

In the second experiment, it was found that allicin and ajoene inhibit the expression of iNOS in activated macrophages (Dirsch *et al.*, 1998b). Since it is known that the inflammatory environment in human atherosclerotic lesions results in the expression of the inducible form of nitric oxide synthase and subsequently in the formation of peroxynitrite, and by this aggravates the atherogenic process, these results may provide an interesting basic contribution with regard to the beneficial effects claimed for garlic in the prophylaxis of atherosclerosis. Meanwhile it has also been shown that the mistletoe lectin I of *Viscum album* is able to induce the apoptosis of cancer cells, suggesting that, in addition to the well-known immunostimulating activity, a second molecular biological mechanism for the described antitumour activity of mistletoe preparations has been found.

These examples, which could be extended by many others (e.g. plant extracts and constituents with calcium-antagonistic, endothelin-inhibiting, COX2-inhibiting, leucotriene-antagonistic, immunomodulating or antifibrotic activity), demonstrate the need to introduce new molecular biological models for the screening of phytopreparations and herbal drug constituents.

Mechanism of action of phytopharmaceuticals

The experience-based claim of phytotherapy that the therapeutic effects of plant extracts or the constituents of herbal drugs are in many cases superior to isolated single compounds from the same plants, or mixtures of them, has never been assessed in systematic pharmacological or clinical studies. There are, however, numerous practical experiences and clinical effects that support this claim. Previous results in classical pharmacology using mixtures of bioactive compounds have shown that differentiation between additive and synergistic over-additive or potentiating effects is necessary. If two substances of a mixture have the same pharmacological target, an additive effect can be expected. If, however, two or more substances of a mixture have different pharmacological targets, a pharmacologically synergistic effect may result that can be greater than that expected for the individual substances taken together (provided none of the substances in the mixture exerts an antagonizing effect). As described in more detail in Chapter 4, such dose–response investigations with mixtures of bioactive compounds can be carried out by using the isobole methods as proposed by Berenbaum (1989). This method has been applied for the rationalization of synergistic effects of mixtures of antiviral compounds (for example, Hall and Duncan, 1988).

The author and colleagues carried out a similar experiment using thrombocyte aggregation assay with a mixture of ginkgolide A and B, two major constituents of *Ginkgo biloba*, and found a typical synergistic effect as shown by the 'concave-up' isobole curve in Figure 3.1 (Steinke, 1993; see also Chapter 4).

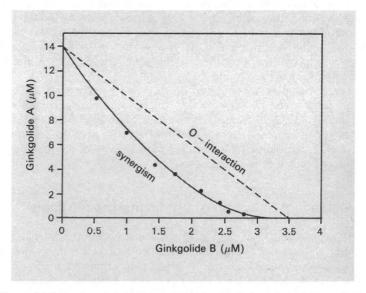

Figure 3.1 Synergism of ginkgolide A and ginkgolide B (isobole method; $n = 2$–9)

It is evident that this isobole method cannot be applied to herbal extracts or mixtures. In this context it may be mentioned that in classical chemotherapy, the application of mixtures of substances (such as the three nucleotides contained in a cocktail for AIDS therapy) has found a striking renaissance. The better overall effect of this triple therapy for AIDS can be explained by a polyvalent or multivalent action of these substances on three distinct target enzymes (reverse transcriptase, protease and glucosidase). The synergistic effects within herbal extracts and multi-herbal preparations has to be interpreted in a similar way.

In discussing the possible molecular biological mechanisms of synergistic therapeutic effects, it must be considered that these effects can also partly be explained by an enhanced absorption rate and better bioavailability caused by non-bioactive constituents of the same herbal drug, such as tannins or saponins. On the other hand, many controlled clinical studies of standardized phytopreparations are available which verify the hypothesis of synergistic effects of bioactive constituents within herb extracts and drug combinations. The therapeutically used ginkgo and St John's wort phytopreparations may support this hypothesis. For the generation of a PAF-antagonizing effect in humans, about 100–240 mg of a standardized ginkgolide A, B, C mixture per day must be administered (Chung *et al.*, 1988). The same effect can be achieved by a daily dose of 120 mg of standardized ginkgo extract containing altogether about 6–7 mg of ginkgolides, bilobalide and flavonol-glycosides. Obviously, this low concentration of ginkgo constituents in the ginkgo extract is bioequivalent to 100–240 mg pure ginkgolides. A similar calculation might be valid for St. John's wort (*Hypericum perforatum*) extracts. One of the last clinical trials performed with standardized Hypericum extracts against synthetic Imipramin for 'moderate depression' resulted, after 6 weeks' treatment, in the same reduction of the depression score values on the HAMDA depression scale (Vorbach *et al.*, 1993). It appears that 900 mg of Hypericum extract applied per day, containing altogether about 8–10 mg bioactive compounds (hypericines, hyperforins, flavonoids, procyanidins), can be regarded as bioequivalent to 75 mg synthetic Imipramin.

This comparison of bioequivalence leads to the conclusion that phytotherapy (with some exceptions) is a low-dose therapy in relation to the amount of applied bioactive compounds of a plant extract. In terms of classical pharmacology, this low concentration of active compounds could be classified as 'underdosage'. The successful results obtained with phytopreparations in controlled clinical trials, however, disprove this opinion. A recently performed investigation of mistletoe strengthens the low-dose hypothesis.

Mistlelectine I, the presumed major active substance of *Viscum album* extracts, stimulates the cytokine production and phagocytic activity of macrophages in breast cancer patients, and by this the overall immune response, at the surprisingly low concentration of 1 ng/kg (i.v. or i.m.) (Hajto *et al.*, 1989).

A scientific explanation is lacking for these synergistic and low-dose phenomena. The frequently observed reverse effects of bioactive compounds, if they are used once in a high and then in a very low concentration, also cannot be rationalized. Experiments carried out by the author and colleagues with classical cytostatic agents of natural and synthetic origin such as vincristine, taxol, podophyllotoxin, naphthoquinones, methotrexate or fluoruracil are particularly impressive. When used in subtoxic amounts (μg or pg range), *in vitro* granulocyte or T-lymphocyte assays showed immunostimulatory effects. In high concentrations (mg), the known cytostatic, cytotoxic or immunosuppressive activity occurred (Wagner *et al.*, 1988).

Another as yet unresearched area of phytotherapy is the phenomenon of the increasing effects of phytopreparations during the course of long-term therapy administered at low doses. Measurements of myocardial blood perfusion in dogs using a thermoprobe led, following a 3-week course of very low doses of Crataegus extracts, to a maximum blood supply (three to four times higher than on day 0 of administration). This result was only evident after 3 weeks' treatment, and agrees with the subjective results noted by patients in clinical trials (Mävers and Hensel, 1974).

Observations that very low doses result in an effect after reaching a threshold concentration have until now only been shown in plant physiology.

Conclusion

The polyvalent activity and the observed synergistic effects exerted by many phytopreparations need to be more closely studied by intensive target-directed pharmacological investigations using new molecular biological models. Efforts should also be made to clarify the unsolved questions concerning the proper dosages of phyto-preparations, the mechanism of long-term effects and the phenom-enon of dose-dependent pharmacological reverse effects.

References

Bauer, R. and Tittel, G. (1996). Quality assessment of herbal preparations as a precondition of pharmacological and clinical studies. *Phytomedicine*, 2, 193–8.

Berenbaum, M. C. (1989). What is synergy? *Pharmacol. Rev.*, 41, 93.

Chung, P., Brambilla, C., Duhier, J. *et al.* (1988). Chapt. 4, In *Ginkgolides – Chemistry, Pharmacology and Clinical Perspectives* (P. Braquet, ed.), pp. 345–54. J. R. Prous Science Publ.

Dirsch, V. M., Gerbes, A. L. and Vollmar, A. M. (1998a). Ajoene, a compound of garlic, induces apoptosis in human promyeloic cells, accompanied by generation of reactive oxygen species and activation of nuclear factor κB. *Molecular Pharmacol.*, 53, 402–7.

Dirsch, V. M., Kiemer, A. K., Wagner, H. and Vollmar, A. M. (1998b). Effect of allicin and ajoene, two compounds of garlic, on inducible nitric oxide synthase. *Atherosklerosis*, 139, 333–9.

ESCOP (1993). *Notice to Applicants for Marketing Authorisation for Medicinal Products for Human Use in the Member States of the European Communities*, Vol. IIA. European Scientific Co-operative of Phytotherapy.

Franck, U., Günther, B., Vierling, W. and Wagner, H. (1996) Investigation of *Cecropia* and *Crataegus* extracts for their angiotensin-converting enzyme inhibitory and vasorelaxant activities *Phytomedicine*, 1, 93.

Geiger, W. N. (1998). Studien zur p.o. Bioverfügbarkeit von *Urtica dioica* – Agglutinin (UDA) und Untersuchungen von UDA und anderen Lektinen zur Wirkung auf Wachstumsfaktoren und Tyrosinphosphorylierung, Thesis, Munich University.

German Commission E at the FR-German Health Authority (Berlin) and Keller, K. (1991). *J. Ethnopharmacol.*, 32, 225–9.

Hajto, T., Hostanka, K. and Gabius, H. J. (1989) Modulatory potency of the β-galactoside specific lectin from mistletoe extract (Iscador) on the host defense system *in vivo* in rabbits and patients. *Cancer Res.*, 49, 4803–8.

Hall, M. J. and Duncan, I. B. (1988). Chapt. 8, In *Antiviral Agents: The Development and Assessment of Antiviral Chemotherapy* (H. J. Field, ed.), Vol. II, pp. 29–84. CRC Press Boca Raton.

IFPMA (1997). Major steps towards global drug regulations (4 ICH Conference in Brussels). *Health Horizons*, 32.

Mävers, W. H. and Hensel, H. (1974). Veränderungen der lokalen Myokard-durchblutung nach oraler Gabe eines Crataegus-Extraktes bei nicht narkotisierten Hunden. *Arzneim. Forsch.*, 24, 783.

Peumans, W. J., De-Ley, M. and Broehaert, W. F. (1984) An unusual lectin from stinging nettle (*Urtica dioica*) rhizomes. *FEBS Lett.*, 177, 99–103.

Schilcher, H. (1998). Herbal drugs in the treatment of benign prostatic hyperplasia. In *Phytomedicines of Europe* (L. D. Lawson and R. Bauer, eds). American Chemical Society Symposium Series 691.

Steinke, B. (1993). Chemisch-analytische und pharmakologische Untersuchungen von pflanzlichen PAF-Antagonisten und Inhibitoren der Thrombozytenaggregation (Allium-Arten, *Ginkgo biloba, Pinellia ternata*). Thesis, Munich University.

Tauchert, M., Bloch, M. and Hübner, W. D. (1994). Wirksamkeit des Weißdorn-Extraktes LI 132 imVergleich mit Captopril-Multizentrische

Doppelblindstudie bei 192 Patienten mit Herzinsuffizienz im Stadium II nach NYHA. *Münch. Med. Wschr.*, **136**(Suppl. 1), 27.

Vorbach, E. H., Hübner, W. D. and Arnoldt, K. H. (1993) Wirksamkeit und Verträglichkeit des Hypericum Extraktes LI 160 im Vergleich mit Imipramin, *Nervenheilkunde*, **12**, 290–96.

Wagner, H., Kreher, B. and Jurcic K. (1988). *In vitro* stimulation of human granulocytes and lymphocytes by pico- and femtogram quantities of cytostatic agents. *Arzneim. Forsch.*, **38**, 273–5.

Wagner, H., Elbl, G., Lotter, H. and Guinea, M. (1991) Evaluations of natural products as inhibitors of angiotensin-I-converting enzyme (ACE). *Pharm. Pharmacol. Lett.*, **1**, 15–18.

Wagner, H., Willer, F., Samtleben, R. and Boos, G. (1994) Search for the antiprostatic principle of stinging nettle (*Urtica dioica*) roots. *Phytomedicine*, **1**, 213–14.

Wagner, H., Geiger, W. N., Boos, G. and Samtleben, R. (1995) Studies on the binding of *Urtica dioica* agglutinin (UDA) and other lectins in an *in vitro* epidermal growth factor receptor test. *Phytomedicine*, **4**, 287–90.

WHO (1991). Drug regulatory authorities. *Report of the Conference Proceedings, Ottawa, Canada from 7–11 October 1991*, pp. 73–80. WHO.

4

Synergy – myth or reality?

E. M. Williamson

Introduction

Synergy is normally assumed to play a part in the medicinal effects of herbal extracts, and is considered to be one of the great assets of phytotherapy. By synergy, we usually mean that some kind of moderation of activity between the ingredients is taking place, which may be either a potentiation of beneficial effects or an attenuation of undesirable effects (which would more correctly be termed antagonism, but the result should be therapeutically advantageous). The term synergy is unfortunately often used rather loosely and intended to include all kinds of interaction between constituents of a single extract, as well as the components of a multiple herbal mixture.

It is almost inescapable that these interactions between ingredients will occur; however, whether the effects are truly synergistic or merely additive is open to question, and in fact precise evidence for either is very difficult to find. This is surprising given the popularity of products such as those containing garlic, hypericum, ginkgo, valerian and ginseng extracts, where attempts are rarely made to isolate a single constituent; and the ever-increasing interest in traditional Chinese medicine and Ayurveda, where combinations of herbs are routine. Medical herbalists have always ascertained that they obtain superior results with whole extracts rather than with isolated compounds from the same plant; for example, the side effects of ephedrine are not usually found with an extract of ephedra. If true synergy is occurring in these preparations it is important that we should know that this is the case, as it affects the way we use and standardize them. Differences in the ratio between *synergistic* agents are important and variations in the ratio may make results unpredictable, whereas if *additive* effects are the case the ratio is less crucial and effects more predictable. It may therefore be useful to define *synergy* more specifically and to use the term *polyvalent action* when we are unsure of the nature of the interaction, or when the net effect depends on various kinds of constituents although they are not necessarily synergistic.

What is synergy?

Synergy broadly means 'working together', and antagonism 'working against each other', although these terms are ambiguous and imply a quantitative criterion. Obviously, we would consider synergy to be occurring when the combined action of two or more constituents is greater than we would expect from a consideration of the individual contribution of each taken together. Antagonism is easier to define as a reduction in the expected effect. Although the idea of synergy is easy to grasp, the measurement of it is not, as will be explained. It is fairly straightforward identifying synergy when one of the agents is inactive in the system under study, and a combination of this with an active agent produces an effect greater than that observed for the active alone. However, difficulties in measurement arise when both (and of course there may be many more than two) are active. There is still confusion as to how this should be calculated, and various means are available. These have been explained thoroughly by Berenbaum (1989), but the most commonly used are illustrated briefly below.

Summation of effects

If the total effect of a combination is greater than would be expected from the sum of effects, synergy is often the conclusion. This can be expressed mathematically as

$$E(d_a, d_b) = E(d_a) + E(d_b)$$

where d_a and d_b are the doses of a and b.

The validity of this method would appear to be self-evident, but in fact it depends upon the mechanism of action being similar for both agents, and assumes linearity of response, which may not be the case. The method is valid under such conditions, but with herbal mixtures it is unlikely to be appropriate, especially using complex mixtures.

Measurement of the effect of a fixed dose of one on the dose–response curve of the other

This again assumes a knowledge of the dose–response curve of each agent and linearity of response, and would almost certainly be impossible with a complex herbal mixture.

Comparison of the effect of a combination with that of each of its constituents

This was an early method suggested by Gaddum (1940). Synergy was deemed present if the effect of a combination exceeded that of each of its constituents (i.e. d_a, d_b d_a, and d_a, d_b d_b), and antagonism occurred when the effect of one component resulted in a reduction in the effect of another. Although this appears reasonable at first sight (and is at least independent of a knowledge of the mechanism of action), it can be seen to be flawed by considering the case of a sham combination (where a and b are the same agent and interaction cannot therefore occur). Berenbaum quotes the argument of Smith *et al.* (1987) to demolish this method effectively: if two men working separately can cut down 10 trees in a day but working together they cut down 15, then they are certainly not 'working together' – quite the opposite – but the effect of the combination exceeds that of each constituent and would actually fulfil Gaddum's criteria. This method is therefore valid only for antagonism, and is no longer used.

The isobole method

Although this is theoretically the most complicated, it should be the method of choice and is particularly suited to the analysis of effects in herbal mixtures because it is independent of any knowledge of mechanisms and applies under almost all conditions. It makes no assumptions about the behaviour of the components and is also applicable to multiple mixtures. An isobole is an 'iso-effect' curve, in which a combination of ingredients (d_a, d_b) is represented by a point on a graph, the axes of which are the dose axes of the individual agents (D_a and D_b). If agents do not interact, the isobole (the line joining the points representing the combination to those on the dose axes representing the individual doses iso-effective with the combination) will be a straight line. If synergy is occurring (i.e. the combination is more effective than expected from their dose–response curves), then smaller amounts are needed to produce the effect whilst the individual doses remain the same, and the isobole is said to be 'concave-up' (Figure 4.1). The opposite applies for antagonism, producing a 'concave-down' isobole (Figure 4.2).

For one- or two-dose combinations the following equations can be used, showing that although the method is a little difficult in theory, it is fairly convenient in practice:

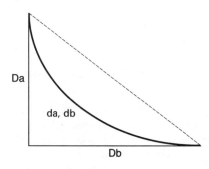

Figure 4.1 Effect of synergy: the 'concave-up' isobole. Da and Db are the individual doses of a and b; da and db are the doses of a and b in the mixture. The dashed line shows zero interaction, i.e. all combination doses to produce this effect if no interaction occurs. Synergy is shown by the solid curve.

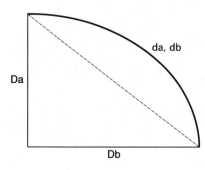

Figure 4.2 Effect of antagonism: the 'concave-down' isobole. Da and Db are the individual doses of a and b; da and db are the doses of a and b in the mixture. The dashed line shows zero interaction. Antagonism is shown by the solid curve.

The equation for *zero interaction* is $\dfrac{da}{Da} + \dfrac{db}{Db} = 1$

So the expression for *synergy* must be $\dfrac{da}{Da} + \dfrac{db}{Db} < 1$

(i.e. smaller amounts of a and/or b are needed to produce the same effect),

and the expression for *antagonism* is $\dfrac{da}{Da} + \dfrac{db}{Db} > 1$

(i.e. larger amounts of a and/or b are needed to produce the same effect).

It can be seen from these that it is not always necessary to have complete dose–response curves to demonstrate synergy with this method (although it is possible to have synergy at a particular dose combination with antagonism at a different combination, which should be borne in mind). Antagonism is just as important, as one of the main tenets of herbalism holds that toxicity of plant extracts is to be less than that of a single compound resulting in a similar effect, and it can be dealt with in the same way.

Berenbaum also described other approaches to defining synergy (including the most commonly used and erroneous method, whereby criteria are not defined at all), and these, together with examples and proofs of the methods, can be found in his work (Berenbaum, 1989).

Other interactions that could be synergistic or antagonistic *in vivo* but not necessarily *in vitro* are those combinations of ingredients that would either hinder or enhance activity by affecting absorption, metabolism or excretion. Unless a similar reaction actually took place in the test-tube (as, for example, the complexing of polyphenols and tannins with many drugs), then these effects would only be noticeable in the whole organism. In practice, the complexing of tannin-containing drugs in the stomach does not seem to be a real problem, otherwise tea drinkers would find many of their prescribed medications to be clinically ineffective. Empirical effects found with mixtures are at least as important as the results obtained with isolated compounds, and clinical evaluation the most important objective of all.

Polyvalent action

Returning to the idea that a range of active constituents is important in herbal medicine, it is convenient to consider the contribution of different kinds of ingredients to the overall effect of a herb or herb mixture, whether or not they act in true synergy. It is common medical practice to use several drugs to treat a single complaint (e.g. pain, hypertension and especially cancer) and the rationale is equally applicable to plant extracts – in fact more so, since the combinations are already an actuality within the plant. There are also good reasons for not isolating individual components, summarized in Table 4.1, the first of which is probably the 'if it ain't broke, don't fix it' approach, which is normally a good idea in most aspects of life! Therefore, tried and tested herbs such as Echinacea and ginseng, which have been around for centuries, are usually left as they are and total extracts used as a matter of course. This is certainly not an argument against standardization and quality control – it is still important to know the effects of the various types of constituent in order to enable good, reproducible products to be produced, containing known actives, which will ensure consistent therapeutic responses.

Table 4.1 Reasons for not isolating active constituents from plant extracts

Reason	Examples
Extract investigated and accepted *per se*	*Ginkgo biloba*, Echinacea, ginseng
Unsure of active constituent(s)	*Hypericum perforatum*, raspberry leaf
Instability of actives	Garlic, valerian
Synergy/antagonism known or suspected	Kava, *Artemisia annua*, valerian, liquorice

   Another, even more obvious, reason for not isolating compounds is when we do not know exactly what they are. The most important actives of even such a significant herb as St. John's wort are still under discussion, and even if we are unsure that true synergy is occurring, it would be unwise to exclude any of the constituents suspected of contributing to efficacy. In some cases actives are unstable, and attempt to remove them from the 'protection' of the herb or whole extract would be counter-productive. Here the obvious examples are garlic and valerian. Garlic is sometimes presented as a product that contains the 'precursor' alliin and the enzyme allicinase, which in solution (i.e. in the stomach) liberates the active alliin and eventually other, unstable, active, decomposition products. This is certainly not synergy and possibly not polyvalent action either, but is in effect a drug delivery system. There are also instances where the active ingredient has never been properly identified and is suspected of being unstable, such as raspberry leaf (although this may be a perfect example of synergy of course!). Instances of polyvalent action will be dealt with later, using examples of both single and multiple herb extracts.

Synergy in single herb extracts

Demonstrating synergy within a single herbal extract is difficult. It requires fractionation of the extract, testing each component and then putting it all back together again and testing the whole. It is also necessary to test all the permutations of the various isolates to see how each is interacting with the other(s). This is probably why information is so sparse; nevertheless, some data is available to support the view that it happens, although we usually have little idea of how it may be mediated.

Artemisia annua

The Chinese antimalarial herb *Artemisia annua* contains many compounds in addition to artemisinin, a sesquiterpene lactone that has been extracted and used to produce more stable derivatives such as artemether. Both are now in clinical use in various parts of the world. Phillipson (1999) has reported work carried out by his group on the different constituents of this herb, where they discovered that the flavonoids also present significantly enhanced the *in vitro* antimalarial activity of artemisinin against *Plasmodium falciparum*. Although not clinical evidence, it does show that the synergistic activity is not just a question of enhanced absorption, excretion or bioavailability *in vivo*.

Kava

Synergy has also been proposed in the effects of the psychoactive herb kava, *Piper methysticum* (Klohs *et al.*, 1959), which is used in the South Pacific as a sedative, euphoriant and mild hallucinogen, and as part of various religious rites. A crude extract of ground kava root and several isolated known sedative compounds were each tested for their effects on the central nervous system by determining their ability to antagonize clonic strychnine-induced convulsions and death in mice. The total extract was particularly effective, and dihydromethysticin (DHM) was found to be the most potent individual component. A mixture of kawain, dihydrokawain, methysticin, dihydromethysticin, yangonin and dihydroyangonin, in the same ratio in which they were found in the crude extract, was then tested and related to a potency similar to that of DHM. However, as this compound represented only 5 per cent of the total extract, and the other constituents were known to be less potent than DHM, the mixture was deemed synergistic. This is further substantiated by Meyer (1967), who reported that the anticonvulsant action of yangonin and desmethoxyyangonin is increased when given with other kava constituents, measured as prevention of maximum electric shock seizure. Further details of the complex pharmacology of kava are available in the review by Singh and Blumenthal (1997).

Valerian

Valerian is a widely used sedative herb, and it is well known that several different types of compounds present in it have sedative activity. The nature of the interactions which may be occurring is not fully known, but there is some evidence that synergism is present. Holzl (1997, and references therein) reported that an extract of *Valeriana officinalis* reduces glucose consumption in areas of the rat brain, especially the cortex and limbic system; however, the isolated single substances valtrate, didrovaltrate, valerenic acid and valerenone showed no such effect, although they are known to be sedative in other biological systems. This may be because the researchers did not identify the actual compound responsible for the activity, or it may be an indication that synergism is occurring.

Liquorice

A small study on the bioavailability of glycyrrhizin when given on its own or as part of a liquorice root extract has shown that absorption of glycyrrhizin is lower when taken in the form of the extract than if given alone (Cantelli-Forti *et al.*, 1994). Liquorice (*Glycyrrhiza glabra*) is used for many purposes that do not necessarily depend on its glycyrrhizin content, such as for flavouring as well as for its anti-ulcer, anti-inflammatory, antihepatotoxic and phytoestrogenic effects. Although glycyrrhizin may be active in some of these respects, other components such as the flavones, isoflavones and chalcones are also active, and glycyrrhizin is certainly responsible for some of the more serious side effects associated with ingestion of large amounts of liquorice. Monitoring of blood and urine levels in volunteers who had ingested glycyrrhizin either alone or as an equivalent dose in liquorice showed significantly lower levels in those who had taken the extract. Although the sample size was small (eight people), when a similar experiment was carried out in rats, the results were in agreement. The authors suggested that differences were due to some (unspecified) interaction that takes place during intestinal absorption. Liquorice also features as a synergist in some multi-herbal preparations and as an antagonist in cases of toxicity associated with other herbs, and these will be discussed separately.

Other miscellaneous synergistic interactions

Quillaia saponin adjuvant

Saponins are surfactants with biological activity, and it is not unexpected that they will have modifying effects on other agents given concurrently. *Quillaia saponaria* saponins are used as adjuvants in ISCOM (ImmunoStimulating COMplex) vaccines, where they enhance the antibody response to an antigen (Bomford, 1988, and references therein). At present they are more widely used in veterinary medicine. It is likely that other saponin-containing drugs have a similar effect as well as additional, as yet not defined, synergistic activity.

Dragon's blood
In some cases a single plant extract could be described as exhibiting synergism in that several components are necessary for the action, although it may not be true synergy. The sap of *Croton draconoides* and *C. lechleri*, also known as dragon's blood because of its dark red, viscous nature, is used topically to aid wound healing. These properties are thought to be due to various fractions of the sap – for example, the occlusive action of the sap dries to form a semipermeable covering over a wound, and within this protective layer the polyphenols act to prevent ingress of external microbes. The anti-inflammatory and antioxidant compounds also present in the sap will contribute to the healing and protective action (Chen *et al.*, 1994).

Antioxidants
Many natural products have free radical or antioxidant activity, which would contribute to a number of biological activities such as anti-inflammatory effects. One of these is apocynin, from *Picrorhiza kurroa*, which also inhibits NF-κB dependent release of tumour necrosis factor (TNF). This has been proposed as a useful property for the adjunctive treatment of viral diseases, since NF-κB is considered to be an important mediator of viral expresion in HIV-infected subjects (Beukelman *et al.*, 1995). Flavonoids and polyphenolics have antioxidant properties, which could lead to modulatory or synergistic activity in many mixtures, and may well act as modifiers (or synergists) in many conditions. They are presently the subject of intensive research.

Synergy in multi-herb preparations

It is the general rule rather than the exception that herbalists use mixtures of extracts, designed to give the best therapeutic outcome with minimal side effects. Many traditional prescriptions are historical combinations, and evidence as to the importance of their exact constitution is lacking although their efficacy is not in question. Combinations of herbs are used to 'fine tune' the organism rather than hit a particular biochemical target, and this makes evaluating either additive or synergistic effects even more difficult than usual. Simple examples would be the inclusion of laxative herbs in products used for haemorrhoids, or choleretic herbs in digestive preparations. However, it is at least possible to test the effect of individual extracts singly and in combination and this will give an indication of synergy or antagonism although no real evidence as to which compounds are interacting.

Traditional Chinese medicine

Traditional Chinese medicine (TCM), in particular, uses complicated recipes and unusual methods (to Western thought) of processing extracts. For example, paeony root (*Paeonia lactiflora*) is treated by stir-baking to char, stir-baking with vinegar, steaming with wine and so on, depending on its proposed usage. These processes have been shown to affect the yield of the various components of the extract (Sheu and Han, 1994), and it is therefore important that when studies (including those intended to demonstrate synergy) are done, the preparation method is taken into account. Paeony root is a component of a highly efficacious TCM treatment for eczema, which has been the subject of a clinical trial of 37 young patients (Sheehan and Atherton, 1992). Investigations were carried out to identify the 'active constituent' of the mixture, but a programme of pharmacological and clinical tests showed there was no single active herb or active principle, and that it was the mixture of 10 herbs that was so effective. Apart from paeony, the herbs included *Ledebouriella divaricata*, *Glycyrrhiza uralensis*, *Saposhnikovia divaricata*, *Schizonepeta tenuifolia*, *Rehmannia glutinosa*, *Lophatherum gracile*, *Tribulus terrestris*, *Dictamnus dasycarpus*, *Potentilla chinensis* and *Clematis armandii* (Phillipson, 1994).

Liquorice is present in a great many other TCM prescriptions, and the reason for its inclusion is not always immediately apparent, although evidence for its potentiating and detoxifying properties is now emerging. Paeoniflorin, from paeony root, inhibits the twitch responses of skeletal muscle to direct and indirect stimulation at high doses. When given in combination with glycyrrhizin, potentiation of the neuromuscular blocking effect occurs both *in vitro* and *in vivo* (Hikino, 1985, and references therein). In TCM, an extract may be added to a prescription purely to attenuate the side effects of another, and an example is the use of liquorice as a detoxifier. Many Chinese physicians insist on using liquorice (*Radix glycyrrhizae*) in conjunction with aconite root (*Radix aconiti preparata*), and a recent preliminary study has produced some evidence to support this. When the amount of liquorice in the preparation 'Sini decoction' (which contained fixed amounts of aconite and ginger extract) was increased, a corresponding reduction in the amount of aconitine that could be extracted from the decoction was observed (Miaorong and Jing, 1994). This study is not comprehensive in any way, but indicates that the subject of detoxification by use of liquorice deserves further attention. It is quite probable that many of the principles of combinations observed in TCM will be found to be based on similar phenomena, although the experiments needed to prove this are rather daunting in their complexity.

Ayurveda

Ayurveda, arguably the oldest system of medicine in the world, also uses combinations of herbs with set formulations. An important ingredient of many recipes is 'Trikatu' (a Sanskrit word meaning 'three acrids'), which is a mixture of black pepper (*Piper nigrum*), long pepper (*Piper longum*) and ginger (*Zingiber officinalis*). Trikatu is used as an ingredient of numerous prescriptions, some of which date back to 6000 BC. The reason for the inclusion of these same herbs has recently been investigated, and a rationale for their use postulated involving enhancement of bioavailability, by Trikatu but especially by the alkaloid piperine from *Piper nigrum* (Johri and Zutshi, 1992, and references therein). Piperine has been shown in several studies in both humans and animals to increase blood levels of herbal drugs such as vasicine (an anti-asthmatic alkaloid also known as peganine, from *Adhatoda vesica*) as well as rifampicin, theophylline and others. It has been shown that the bioavailability enhancement is probably a result of the fact that piperine is a potent inhibitor of drug metabolism (Atal *et al.*, 1985). The other components of Trikatu have not been investigated in the same way, so it is not known if there is a similar rationale for their use.

European herbalism

In Europe, set formulae for herbal products are also used, with some historical precedence, although generally not as rigidly as in the previous examples. We are now realizing that these empirically derived mixtures often have an efficacy as yet unexplained, since the dose levels of the component herbs often seem too low to have a therapeutic effect. This would, of course, be indicative of synergy. A common formula used to treat benign prostatic hyperplasia (BPH) consists of nettle root (*Urtica dioica*) with pygeum bark (*Pygeum africanum*), sometimes with other herbs. This combination has been shown to have synergistic activity in an *in vitro* system, where its effect against the enzymes aromatase and 5-α-reductase, which are implicated in BHP, were tested. Nettle root extract alone was only effective against either enzyme at high concentrations, and pygeum bark, although more active on 5-α-reductase, had only weak activity against aromatase. The combination showed a potency equivalent to that of pygeum bark on 5-α-reductase, and aromatase was significantly more inhibited by a mixture of the extracts than by each separately (Hartmann *et al.*, 1996).

A mixture of herbs used in Italy to aid digestion, known as Amaro Medicinale Giuliani, has been shown to be clinically effective and the mixture to be more efficacious than the extracts, which were tested in pairs (consisting of gentian + rhubarb and boldo + cascara) against placebo. Although synergy is not quite proven, the ingredients are working together and a case can be made for the inclusion of each: gentian (*Gentiana lutea*) and rhubarb (*Rheum* spp.) both stimulate gastric secretion (at high doses rhubarb is laxative, but in this preparation the dose is low); boldo leaf (*Peumus boldo*) is reputed to increase bile flow; and cascara (*Rhamnus purhiana*) increases colonic peristalsis by stimulating the myoenteric plexus. The mixture was also shown to increase pancreatic exocrine secretion by an unknown mechanism and to accelerate gastro-intestinal motility in humans to a greater extent than the pairs of extracts tested, and it is therefore thought to act as a digestive by stimulating the appetite, aiding gastric, pancreatic and biliary secretions and enhancing colonic transit (Brunetti *et al.*, 1992).

Theoretical interactions within alkaloid-containing plants have been described (Izaddoost and Robinson, 1987), although the evidence produced in this reference does not actually demonstrate the presence of synergy as opposed to additive effects. The lack of conclusive evidence illustrates the difficulties in identifying synergy and supports the use of the more general term, polyvalent action, which is broader and does not exclude synergy should it occur.

Examples of polyvalent action within a single herb extract

The term polyvalent action can be used to describe the effect of multiple active constituents acting in combination, in harmony and possibly in synergy. It therefore overcomes the problems inherent in describing the total effect as synergistic, and can even include antagonism where that applies to undesirable side effects. The vast majority of herbal extracts must work in this way, as very few contain only one active ingredient and all multi-herb products act like this by definition. Many examples can be given, but it is useful to use those that contain at least two different types of chemical compounds with well-defined activities known to contribute to the effect.

Ginkgo biloba
The constituents of *Ginkgo biloba* have been well investigated, and most ginkgo preparations are standardized for concentrations of the

ginkgolides, flavonoids and sesquiterpenes. These groups of compounds have discrete modes of action; however, it is likely that they work together although not necessarily synergistically. Historically ginkgo is used for two main indications, asthma and cerebral insufficiency, and these can be related to the different constituents to some extent.

The ginkgolides are diterpenes with a unique cage-like structure, and are known to be platelet activating factor (PAF) antagonists. PAF is a phospholipid involved in many pathophysiological states, including allergic inflammation, anaphylactic shock and asthma. Many studies over the years have shown that the ginkgolides can antagonize many of the effects of PAF, such as bronchoconstriction, bronchial hyper-responsiveness, platelet aggregation, allergic responses and others. They may contribute to the use of ginkgo in cerebral insufficiency, but their main benefit is probably in inflammatory disorders including asthma (Chung *et al.*, 1987; Newall *et al.*, 1996, and references therein).

Ginkgo flavonoids are known to increase blood circulation to the brain, which is the basis of their use in cerebral insufficiency. Clinical studies have shown ginkgo extracts to be effective in the early stages of dementia, the extract being a total extract not just the flavonoids (Rigney *et al.*, 1999). Current clinical research is showing benefits in all kinds of disorders characterized by impaired cognitive function, and it is likely than the use of ginkgo will increase to even higher levels than at present.

St John's wort

St John's wort (*Hypericum perforatum*) is also one of the most important herbs in clinical use today, and again several constituents of disparate chemical structure are implicated in its action. St John's wort is also another example of a herb containing unstable components, making it unsuitable for fractionation, and here there is some dispute as to the most important class of actives. Its main use is as an antidepressant, but it also has antiviral and wound healing activity.

The hypericins (hypericin, isohypericin and pseudohypericin) are naphthodianthrones, which are photosensitive. They have been reported to have inhibitory activity on monoamine oxidase (MAO) and catechol-O-methyl transferase (COMT), which would substantiate their antidepressant action; however, recently it has been suggested that the *pure* hypericins are either very weak or devoid of activity and positive assay results were due to impurities in the fraction used (Thiede and Walper, 1994). The antidepressant activity may reside in the phloroglucinols (hyperforin and adhyperforin), which is significant because related species of hypericum may not contain them (American Herbal Pharmacopoiea, 1997). Finally, the flavonoids present (especially armentoflavone and bi-apigenin) are sedative and may therefore contribute to activity.

Hypericum extract has been shown to have various biochemical effects associated with antidepressant activity, such as inhibition of serotonin, noradrenaline and dopamine re-uptake, and increasing the number of serotonin receptors (Wheatley, 1998, review). This makes it unique as an antidepressant, but it is not known whether these diverse effects are due to one class of compound or to several, and no evidence is yet available to show whether or not the interaction is synergistic. Therefore, hypericum represents the perfect example of a herb of proven clinical efficacy without the true actives being known, despite the amount of research to which it has been subjected (Wheatley, 1998).

Conclusion

There are numerous other herbs in the same position as St John's wort, where the phytochemistry is well documented but the actual contribution of individual components to the overall effect has not been ascertained (for example, Echinacea spp., *Crataegus oxycantha*, Humulus spp. (hops), *Taraxacum officinale*). It would not be exaggerating to say that this applies to the state of our knowledge of the mode of action of most herbs. Then there are those herbs in use where the phytochemistry is poorly known (*Selenicereus grandiflorus, Symplocarpus foetidus*, etc.) and the pharmacology equally so. If their activity involves synergy (or antagonism) the situation is even more complex, and in this case it is apparent that even bioassay-led fractionation, the normal method used for identifying actives, must be used with caution, since the existence of interactions renders it useless.

In conclusion, there can be no doubt that most herbs rely for their effects on a variety of constituents. Whether they are acting in a truly synergistic way or by additive effects is important mainly for developing methods of standardization, and should be further investigated for this reason, as well as to increase our knowledge of their modes of action. In the meantime, enough evidence is available to show that synergism does occur in herbal extracts and that we should continue to use our whole extracts with confidence, rather than assuming that a single chemical entity is responsible and should be extracted and used alone. Efforts should be directed to ensuring that extracts are standardized properly for the active principles known at the time, and that any synergistic interactions are accommodated where they occur.

References

American Herbal Pharmacopoiea and Therapeutic Compendium (1997). St John's wort, *Hypericum perforatum*. American Herbal Pharmacopoiea.

Atal, C. K., Dubey, R. K. and Singh, J. (1985). Biochemical basis of enhance bioavailability by piperine: evidence that piperine is a potent inhibitor of drug metabolism. *J. Pharm. Exp. Ther.* **232**, 252–258.

Berenbaum, M. (1989). What is synergy? *Pharmacol. Rev.*, **41**, 93–141.

Beukelman, C. J., Van den Berg A. J. J., Kroes, B. H. *et al.* (1995). Plant-derived metabolites with synergistic antioxidant activity. *Immunology Today*, **16**(2), 108.

Bomford, R. (1988). Immunomodulators from plants and fungi. *Phytother. Res.*, **2**, 19–164.

Brunetti, G., Marchioretto, G., Grandinetti, G. *et al.* (1992). Clinical pharmacology of a medicinal herbal digestive complex affecting gastrointestinal functions. In *Natural Drugs and the Digestive Tract* (F. Capasso and N. Mascolo, eds), pp. 15–27. EMSI Roma

Cantelli-Forti, G., Maffei, F., Hrelia, P. *et al.* (1994). Interaction of licorice on glycyrrhizin pharmacokinetics. *Environ. Health Perspect.*, **102**(Suppl. 9), 65–8.

Chen, Z.-P., Cai, Y. and Phillipson, J. D. (1994). Studies on the wound healing properties of Dragon's blood. *Planta Medica*, **60**, 541–5.

Chung, K. F., McCusker, M., Page, P. *et al.* (1987). Effect of a ginkgolide mixture (BN 52063) in antagonising skin and platelet responses to platelet activating factor in man. *Lancet*, **i**, 248–50.

Gaddum, J. H. (1940). *Pharmacology*. Oxford University Press.

Hartmann, R. W., Mark, M. and Soldati, F. (1996). Inhibition of a 5a-reductase and aromatase by PHL-00801 (Prostatonin), a combination of PY 102 (*Pygeum africanum*) and UR 102 (*Urtica dioica*) extracts. *Phytomedicine*, **3/2**, 121–8.

Hikino, H. (1985). Recent research on Oriental medicinal plants. In *Economic and Medicinal Plant Research* (H. Wagner, H. Hikino and N. R. Farnsworth, eds), Vol. 1, pp. 53–85. Academic Press.

Holzl, J. (1997). The pharmacology and therapeutics of *Valeriana*. In *Medicinal and Aromatic Plants – Industrial Profiles* (P. J. Houghton, ed.), Vol 1, pp. 55–75. Harwood Academic Publishers.

Izaddoost, M. and Robinson, T. (1987). Synergy and antagonism in the pharmacology of alkaloidal plants. In *Herbs, Spices and Medicinal Plants: Recent Advances in Botany, Horticulture and Pharmacology* (L. E. Craker and J. E. Simon, eds), Vol. 2, pp. 137–58. Oryx Press.

Johri, R. K. and Zutshi, U. (1992). An Ayurvedic formulation 'Trikatu' and its constituents (review). *J. Ethnopharmacol.*, **37**, 85–91.

Klohs, M. W., Keller, F., Williams, R. E. *et al.* (1959). A chemical and pharmacological investigation of *Piper methysticum* Forst. *J. Med. Pharm. Chem.*, **1**, 95–9.

Meyer, H. J. (1967). Pharmacology of kava. In *Ethnopharmacologic Search for Psychoactive Drugs* (D. H. Efron, B. Holmstedt and N. S. Kline, eds), pp. 133–40. US Dept. of Health, Education and Welfare, Publ. No. 1645, Government Printing Office.

Miaorong, P. and Jing, L. (1996). Correlativity analysis on detoxifying effect of *Radix glycyrrhizae* on *Radix aconiti preparata* in Sini decoction. In *Proc. 40th Ann. Conf.*, Beijing University of Chinese Medicine, August 1996, pp. 28–30. Beijing University Press.

Newall, C. A., Anderson, L. A. and Phillipson, J. D. (1996). Ginkgo. In *Herbal Medicines. A Guide for Healthcare Professionals*, pp. 138–40. Pharmaceutical Press.

Phillipson, J. D. (1994). Traditional medicine treatment for eczema: experience as a basis for scientific acceptance. *Eur. Phytotelegram*, **6**, 33–40.

Phillipson, J. D. (1999). New drugs from plants – it could be yew. *Phytotherapy Res.*, **13**, 1–7.

Rigney, U., Kimber, S. and Hindmarch, I. (1999). The effects of acute doses of standardized *Gingko biloba* extract on memory and psychomotor performance in volunteers. *Phytother. Res.* **13**(1), 408–415.

Sheehan, M. P. and Atherton, D. J. (1992). A controlled trial of traditional Chinese medicinal plants in widespread non-exudative atopic eczema. *Br. J. Dematol*, **126**, 179–184.

Sheu, S.-J. and Han, Y.-J. (1994). A comparative study on processed *Radix Paeoniae Alba. Chinese Pharm. J.*, **46**, 565–73.

Singh, Y. N. and Blumenthal, M. (1997). Kava: an overview. *Herbalgram*, **39**, 33–56.

Smith, G. H., Williams, F. L. R. and Lloyd, O. L. (1987). Respiratory cancer and air pollution from iron foundries in a Scottish town: an epidemiological and environmental study. *Br. J. Indust. Med.*, **44**, 795–802.

Thiede, H.-M. and Walper, A. (1994). Inhibition of MAO and COMT by hypericum extracts and hypericin. *J. Geriatr. Psychiatr. Neur.*, **7**(Suppl. 1), 54–6.

Wheatley, D. (1998). Hypericum extract. Potential in the treatment of depression. *CNS Drugs*, **9**, 431–40.

5

Quality and standardization of herbal medicinal products

D. Loew and A. Schroedter

Introduction

Herbal medicinal products are complex matters; their substantial nature is determined through both the raw materials and the process of preparation (Deutsche Pharmazeutische Gesellschaft, 1998; Gaedcke, 1991). As these parameters can be standardized using modern analytical methods, finished products of constant quality can now be manufactured. With such standardized products, clinical studies can be conducted; however, it must be remembered that there are limitations in the transferability of the results to other products from the same herbal drug (Loew, 1997). As there is no question that the activity of these drugs is based on their constituents, the quality of a preparation is decisive. In this context, the question of comparability or 'essential similarity' of herbal preparations becomes important. Proper regulations are necessary to avoid future fraud and safety problems.

Quality and regulatory authorities

Pharmaceutical issues

The different EC Directives 65/65 EWG, 75/318 EWG and 75/319 EWG provide the basis for national and international marketing authorization. The manufacturer must provide evidence-based or appropriate scientific information concerning the quality, efficacy and safety of the product. In Europe, the pharmaceutical quality of herbal medicinal products has been researched through the activities of the *ad hoc* working group of the European Agency for the Evaluation of Medicinal Products (1999). The result of this work is a comprehensive collection of statements and recommendations regarding the material quality of herbal medicinal products. In a notice to applicants regarding Part 1 of the amendment of EC

Directive 75/318, certain definitions are given regarding quality assurance in herbal preparations:

1. Characterization according to the nature:
   - the relationship betwen the plant raw material and the preparation made from the herbal medicinal product
   - the physical form of the plant-derived preparation (e.g. dry extract)
   - the solvent or solvent mixture (e.g. 60 per cent ethanol v/v).
2. Characterization according to the amount of active principle:
   - the amount of extract present in the pharmaceutical form
   - the amount of the product containing a defined amount of the active principle.

These definitions include:

- Quantities of herbs or preparations
- An exact description of the preparation process
- Control of the starting material (herb or herbal preparation, respectively)
- Details of analytical controls during the preparation process
- Controls of the finished product
- The stability of the product.

For example, the ratio of herbal drug in the preparation itself has to be declared (e.g. *Sennae folium* ethanolic (60 per cent) dry extract (8 : 1); 125 mg dry extract corresponding to 1000 mg *Sennae folium*). The type of the solvent and or solvent mixture characteristics has to be specified (e.g. 60 per cent ethanol v/v), and the physical form (e.g. dry powder or liquid) has to be stated.

With such formal regulatory levels, a good description of the quality of a herbal medicinal product can be achieved.

Efficacy issues

Questions of pharmaceutical quality relate directly to the medicinal value of herbal drugs, as − especially in Germany − generics of well-investigated herbal medicinal products ('phytogenerics') have appeared on the market with increasing frequency, even marketed by pharmaceutical companies, which are known for innovative synthetic compounds. This raises the question of the comparability of such drugs; in clinical terms, do such phytogenerics have therapeutic equivalence? The basic answer to this question is 'yes', provided that 'essential similarity' can be assumed.

A comparison: 'essential similarity' of chemically defined drugs

Only biopharmaceutical *in vitro* and pharmacokinetic *in vivo* equivalence guarantees identical clinical effects. For chemical drugs to be essentially similar, they must fulfil the following criteria of biopharmaceutical identity:

- They must contain the same active ingredients
- They must have the same qualitative and quantitative composition
- There must be the same ratio between active substance and extraction
- The same formulation must be used
- They must have the same *in vitro* rate in the dissolution test under the same test conditions.

Prerequisites for therapeutic equivalence are as follows (Loew, 1997):

- Direct evidence – the same efficacy and safety in clinical studies
- Direct evidence – the same equivalence in effects, i.e. identical pharmacodynamic effects
- Indirect evidence – confirmation of evidence via surrogates area under the curve, (AUC), maximal plasma concentration (Cmax), and time passed since administration at which plasma concentration maximum occurs, (tmax), located within the 90 per cent confidence limits.

Bioequivalence is assumed if the ratios AUC_{Test}/AUC_{Ref} and $Cmax_{Test}/Cmax_{Ref}$, respectively, are calculated to be located within a 90 per cent confidence interval of the following limits or acceptance ranges: in the case of the ratio $AUC_{Ref/Test}$, an acceptance range of 80–125 per cent (log-transformed) applies; in the case of $Cmax_{Ref/Test}$ the same applies, but the range may vary in specific cases between 70 and 143 per cent (log-transformed). For products without modified release, no evaluation of bioequivalence is neccessary for tmax. Regarding tmax, comparison of the median values with non-parametic tests is sufficient.

'Essential similarity' and herbal medicinal products: possibilities and limitations of biopharmaceutical and bioequivalence studies

With chemically defined drugs, products are essentially similar in their pharmacodynamic properties (or, as the rules governing medicinal products in the European Union say, in *'their effects regarding efficacy and safety'*). However, it is not easy to define whether an equivalence in pharmacokinetic parameters is generally regarded as sufficient. The question is, can these principles be used to prove equivalence of herbal medicinal products, or are special guidelines necessary? Also, what kind of problems may arise when assessing products for their pharmaceutical, biopharmaceutical and bioavailability characteristics? In general, we are faced with the following peculiarities of herbal medicinal products (Loew, 1997):

● A herbal medicinal product from a herbal drug or an extract consists of many substances
● Herbal drugs and their extracts are accepted as being the sum of different pharmacologically (in certain cases even antagonistically or synergistically acting) active substances
● Herbal drugs and their extracts are subjected to natural fluctuations
● The active ingredients determining their efficacy are in many cases not known, thus making confirmation of biopharmaceutical quality difficult
● For the same reason, the demonstration of therapeutical equivalence of compound mixtures in biovailability studies is often not possible.

According to the German authority definition of a herbal extract as a multi-substance mixture from a medicinal plant obtained by extraction of specific parts of the plants and corresponding to the active ingredients in each case, each extract exhibits, qualitatively and quantitatively, a specific content spectrum – therefore an extract is not just any extract. It is true that the composition of a herbal drug may vary according to environmental influences, but the problem caused by this fluctuation when preparing a pharmaceutical standard can generally be solved by selection and preparation.

Pharmaceutical data

As described above, formal pharmaceutical specifications are easy to compare. Questions regarding the substantial constitution of preparations cannot be answered sufficiently.

Key issues regarding the question of essential similarity include:

● The raw material – a complete monograph (usually found in pharmacopoeias or produced by the manufacturer) covering all

specifications of identity, purity (exclusion of toxic contaminants) is required
- The extraction solvents used – the type and concentration of extraction media correlate with the composition of an extract; hydrophilic or lipophilic solvents lead to extracts which differ in their spectrum of compounds
- The preparation or manufacturing process – balanced extraction (maceration) and exhaustive extraction (percolation) give very different results. In addition, many company-specific processes and patents can be found.

Products can be evaluated according to these criteria. There are also analytical means (HPLC fingerprint chromatograms) of checking for these substantial basics, as well as for batch-to-batch conformity.

Biopharmaceutical data and herbal medicinal products

As herbal medicinal products have complex constituents, the question of essential similarity between extracts poses additional problems not only on a regulatory level, but also when toxicological, pharmacological and clinical reference to a certain herbal product is made (i.e. using the direct evidence of another product as a type of indirect evidence). Transferring the principles of biopharmaceutical evaluation used for chemical products, the following criteria for herbal products must be fulfilled:

- They must have the same extract or extract fractions, respectively
- There must be the same ratio of herbal drug to extract
- The chemical composition must be the same both in quality and quantity
- There must be the same ratio of active components and extraction
- They must have the same application
- The single and daily dosage must be the same
- The qualitative and quantitative spectrum of constituents *in vitro* must be the same

With analytical means, most questions concerning biopharmaceutical data can be answered. However, some restrictions exist as a consequence of the complex matter being dealt with; individual constituents must be selected, which then act as descriptors of the whole extract. This has to be taken into account when talking about standardization or standardized extracts.

Up to now, no single herbal drug has been identified in which 100 per cent of the extract is characterized with respect to all constituents. Presently, characterization of extracts focuses on compounds, which comprise about 20–30 per cent of the total composition.

Bioequivalence and herbal medicinal products

The search for indirect evidence via bioequivalence studies with herbal drugs is a logical step in cases where evidence is required. It has to be stated that the idea makes sense only when the product itself is strictly defined and manufactured according to standardized procedures with standardized raw materials. Scientifically, it must be remembered that, with herbal drugs, the extract as a whole (and therefore a number of compounds) constitutes 'the active principle' as a whole. Thus, measurement of one or more selected components used as markers is burdened with all the drawbacks of measuring surrogate endpoints.

The question of which constituents are active has been studied sufficiently only in a few herbal drugs. Well-known examples include *Aesculus hippocastanum*, *Piper methysticum* and *Silybum marianum*. Thus, bioavailability and bioequivalence studies are possible. However, in these herbs it is not one single constituent that is active but rather a group of substances of similar structure. This may lead to specific analytical problems if immunological methods must be used due to low concentrations of the constituents of interest. The following example illustrates this.

Extracts from horse-chestnut seeds, standardized to 16–20 per cent of aescin, are used to treat venous insufficiency. A controlled clinical study showed significant results for a specific preparation, which was then used as reference in several bioequivalence studies, all analysed in the same laboratory. Five single-dose and four multiple-dose studies versus different test preparations were conducted, some of them with the result of bioequivalence, others not. Comparing the results of the multiple-dose studies (which are the relevant ones, for the reference preparation only), the data showed only poor reproducibility for the reference drug itself. In one study against a test preparation, where bioequivalence could not be found, the extracts were analysed thoroughly with regard to both their relevant constituents (aescins) and their biopharmaceutical specifications. The latter were comparable regarding total aescin, but the extracts showed major differences for the spectrum of the different aescins. This led to the conclusion that the radioimmunological assay, which was validated with a specific b-aescin, did not react in a similar way to both extracts. The fact that concentrations under steady-state conditions differed markedly before intake of the medication supports the hypothesis that extract-specific validation, especially with immunological assays, is an important issue (Schroedter *et al.,* 1998; Loew *et al.,* 1999).

A careful and considered use of bioavailability/bioequivalence data is necessary when important questions (such as regulatory queries) have to be answered. There are other examples where ongoing research has led to new information about the active principles; however, in most cases the active ingredients are unknown and the herbal drugs are standardized on markers alone. Markers are chemically defined substances that are used for control purposes, and serve to calculate the quantity of herbal drug or preparation in the finished product. No inference from identical markers to equivalents of extracts is permissible. A typical example is *Hypericum perforatum*, one of the most popular herbal drugs. *Hypericum perforatum* is currently being investigated to determine its active ingredients. Most preparations of hypericum are standardized using hypericin as the marker, since the compound hypericin was accepted as being responsible for the antidepressive effects. However, it has since been demonstrated that hyperforin also has relevant activities *in vitro* and *in vivo*, and this question is currently being addressed in pharmacological and clinical studies. The available evidence to date is inconclusive, and expert opinions on this differ considerably.

Data from other drugs (e.g. *Agnus castus*) indicate that a small number of constituents have similar binding characteristics to the dopamine D2 receptor, which means that this group of similar compounds may be responsible for the dopaminergic effect of *Agnus castus* preparations. These examples show that extracts contain several active principles and the overall effect has to be regarded as the result of a complex interaction between the constituents of the extract and the body. Using markers is no solution for this problem. They may well allow us to calculate the total amount of a herbal drug in an extract *in vitro*, but they will show a specific and individual behaviour *in vivo*.

The new draft note for guidance on the investigation of bioavailability and bioequivalence (The Committee for Proprietary Medicinal Products, 1998) rightly states that *in vivo* studies of oral immediate release forms are not necessary if the following criteria are fulfilled:

- The active substance does not have a narrow therapeutic range
- It has a first-pass metabolism > 70 per cent and linear pharmacokinetics within the therapeutic range

- It is highly water soluble
- It is highly permeable in the intestine
- The formulation is not expected to have effects on pharmacokinetic parameters.

For herbal medicinal products these data are usually not available, and it is also not possible to conduct scientifically valid bioequivalence studies for the majority of herbal studies at present. Such studies are not impossible, but even with modern analytical means they still represent a challenge (De Smet and Brouwers, 1997). It must be remembered that data concerning the bioavailability of a selected component carry only information on the behaviour of this component; if this component is a pharmacologically active component the relevance of the information is high, but it is just part of the unknown truth. In every case, the understanding of the pharmacodynamic actions of the botanical drug improves with such data.

Besides the indirect evidence of therapeutic equivalence between herbal drugs, the assessment of the bioavailability of the constituents of a herbal preparation can give valuable information on the activities of a herb, especially on the applicability of pharmacodynamic data of specific compounds which were generated in *in vivo* assays. If the substance is present in reasonable amounts, its *in vitro* properties will come into effect. One example is the immense research carried out with Phyto-SERMs, herbs that contain selective estrogen receptor modulators (SERMs).

Issues to consider concerning essential similarity of herbal medicinal products

The phytogeneric is only comparable to the standard preparation under the following conditions:

- Pharmaceutical equivalence – i.e. raw material quality, extraction, manufacturing process, standardization
- Biopharmaceutical equivalence – i.e. the same extract/extract fractions, the same presentation, the same single and daily dose and *in vitro* qualitative and quantitative conformity
- *In vivo* equivalence in bioequivalence studies.

With modern analytical methods, pharmacokinetic studies of a single compound or several compounds from a herbal drug are still a challenge but are not impossible. Therapeutic equivalence can be assumed in the same way as with chemically defined substances.

However, if pharmaceutical, biopharmaceutical and *in vivo* equivalence studies are not possible, other investigations are necessary:

- Experimental investigations of the pharmacological profile, e.g. *in vitro* in cell-cultured isolated receptor systems, enzymes, isolated organs and in the whole animal
- Clinical-pharmacological investigations on pharmacodynamics
- Clinical investigation on dose and time effect.
- Controlled clinical studies in accordance with the accepted guidelines on clinical efficacy and safety.

Herbal drugs and their preparations are subject to natural variations with respect to their constituents, and may differ in their spectrum of constituents even if the total amount of active principles is constant. From the authors' studies it is known that context or matrix effects may pose problems, especially with immunological assays. Specific validation with respect to the preparations used in the study is necessary to overcome such difficulties (Schroedter *et al.*, 1999).

The activity of herbal medicinal products is not represented by a single constituent. For some herbs, selected constituents can be used based on an informed guess as to their role. Markers as surrogate substances can be used, but it must be remembered that the information on their pharmacokinetic behaviour cannot be extrapolated to the other known or unknown active constituents of the extract.

Conclusion

The quality of herbal medicinal products determines the pharmacodynamic acitivities of the herbal drug and, thus, the therapeutic effects. The list of determinants of the quality of herbal medicinal products is long. Influences from nature are present but, with modern analytical methods and production technology, reproducible herbal medicinal products can be manufactured. In this respect, the situation has fundamentally changed in the last few years, and the old problems with such preparations that led to the isolation and use of single constituents for more predictable effects are resolved.

A complex structure–activity relationship is being suggested. The chances to understand these activities at a microscopic, biochemical level have been improved with new experimental techniques, but the biological total effects of herbal medicinal preparations will probably not be understood if isolated constituents are used as substitutes. The quality of herbal medicinal products has to be checked for a wider spectrum of constituents, taking account of the fact that the relevant ones may still be unknown. In herbal drugs where the active principles are known the situation is not really different, but problems can be resolved because attention can be focused on the relevant substances. From the viewpoint of clinical pharmacology, only the latter herbal medicinal products give the opportunity of studying bioequivalence and thus drawing conclusions of therapeutic equivalence.

For the other herbs, research into the bioavailability of their constituents improves understanding of their possible mechanisms and helps to fill the gaps in current knowledge, which are still wide. High-definition products are needed for such research; as efficacy has been shown for several herbal medicinal products, the challenge of finding the explanation for their success must be addressed. This holds true for clinical pharmacology and for pharmacodynamic activities as well as for interplay between these complex matters.

References

Committee for Proprietary Medicinal Products (1998). Note for guidance on the investigation of bioavailability and bioequivalence. Draft 17.12.1998.

De Smet, P. A. G. M. and Brouwers, J. R. B. J. (1997). Pharmacokinetic evaluation of herbal remedies. *Clin. Pharmacokin.*, **6**, 427–36.

Deutsche Pharmazeutische Gesellschaft (1998). Qualität von Phytopharmaka. DPhG-Symposium Bad Homburg. Deutsche Pharmazeutische Gesellschaft.

EMEA/Herbal Medicinal Products Working Group (1999). Report from the *ad hoc* working group on herbal medicinal products. http://www. eudra. org/emea.html.

Gaedcke, F. (1991). *Phytopharmaka.* Deutsche Apotheker Zeitung (DAZ) **48**: 2551–5.

Loew, D. (1997) Is the biopharmaceutical quality of extracts adequate for clinical pharmacology? *Int. J. Clin. Pharmacol. Ther.*, **35**(7), 302–6.

Loew, D., Schroedter, A., Schwankl, W. and Schneider, B. (1999). The problematic of bio-availablity/bioequivalence of extracts containing β-aescin, a pharmacokinetic review (in preparation).

Schroedter, A., Loew, D., Schwankl, W. and Rietbrock, N. (1998). Zur Validität radioimmunologisch bestimmter Bioverfügbarkeitsdaten von β-Aesin in Rosskastaniensamenextrakten. *Arzn. Forsch.*, **9**, 905–10.

6

The efficacy of herbal drugs

E. Ernst and M. H. Pittler

Introduction

The popularity of herbal remedies is increasing dramatically. Figures relating to the US herbal market, for instance, indicate an increase of 380 per cent in usage between 1990 and 1997 (Eisenberg *et al.*, 1998). *Vis-à-vis* this extraordinary level of popularity, it has therefore become an ethical imperative to determine the efficacy of herbal drugs, i.e. drugs that consist of whole plants, parts of plants or extracts of plants. The accepted 'gold standard' for testing the efficacy of drugs (herbal or synthetic) is the randomized clinical trial. To minimize the influence of patient and therapist expectations, randomized clinical trials of herbal drugs should be conducted double-blind where possible (in some cases this may not be possible; for example, the odour of garlic is likely to 'deblind' such a trial). Depending on the research question, these trials can be conducted against placebo or reference medications (if an efficacious drug for the condition in question exists) or no treatment at all.

However, even rigorous randomized clinical trials do not always agree in their conclusions. A good example is the use of garlic for lowering cholesterol. While most of the early randomized clinical trials were positive (Warshafsky *et al.*, 1993), a number of negative results have recently been published (for example, Berthold *et al.*, 1998). In order to provide a fair estimate of the true overall efficacy of a particular treatment, it is therefore not advisable to rely on data from selected randomized clinical trials. Only the totality of the available data will provide the most reliable evidence and thereby minimize bias and random error.

This aim can be achieved by conducting systematic reviews and meta-analyses (Crombie and McQuay, 1998). The former is a structured and systematic overview on a given subject, which provides a methods section stating all necessary details to guarantee reproducibility. In particular, authors of such publications have to demonstrate that a selective evaluation of randomized clinical trials according to their direction of outcome did not occur and that all the available data that met predefined criteria were taken into account. Meta-analyses represent a sub-species of systematic reviews, which pool data from individual trials and calculate a new overall effect size of a particular outcome measure. The traditional or narrative approach to reviews is today considered obsolete and is burdened with a considerable risk of being misleading. In the following section and in Table 6.1, systematic reviews and meta-analyses on the efficacy of herbal drugs available to date will be summarized. These discussions are necessarily very brief, and the interested reader is referred to the original publications for more details regarding both the methodologies employed and the findings generated.

Herbal drugs

Aloe vera

Aloe vera is popular for topical and systemic applications and is at present promoted for a large variety of conditions. A sizeable body of evidence exists in relation to animal models. A systematic review of all rigorous trials on human patients (Vogler and Ernst, 1999) found some evidence to suggest that it is effective as an adjunct oral treatment for diabetes and dermatological conditions such as herpes and psoriasis. This evidence certainly justifies further research. At present, however, none of the claims made for aloe vera is supported by ultimately compelling data from adequately designed clinical trials.

Artichoke

Several lines of evidence (e.g. *in vitro* experiments, animal studies) suggest that artichoke extracts lower the lipid levels in the blood. Its choleretic properties in particular are well documented. A systematic review of all clinical trials of its effects on serum cholesterol reduction (Pittler and Ernst, 1998a) confirmed the plausibility of this notion. However, only one randomized clinical trial on the subject could be located. It suggested that artichoke extract, administered orally for several weeks, may moderately lower elevated total cholesterol levels in the plasma of patients. It seems essential to have independent replication of these results before accepting artichoke extract as a lipid-lowering agent.

Echinacea

The use of products containing extracts of echinacea for the prevention or the treatment of the common cold is particularly popular in some European countries. A recent Cochrane review (Melchart *et al.*, 1999) including 16 trials with a total of over 3000 participants was, however, inconclusive. The overall result suggests that some echinacea preparations have an effect greater than placebo. Nevertheless, the authors felt that there is insufficient evidence to recommend echinacea extracts for the treatment or prevention of the common cold.

Evening primrose

Premenstrual syndrome is a common disorder, and evening primrose oil is often used to treat its symptoms. Seven placebo-controlled randomized clinical trials were included in a review of the efficacy of evening primrose oil for this condition (Budeiri *et al.*, 1996). The two most rigorous trials did not show beneficial effects beyond placebo. The totality of the current evidence suggests uncertain value of evening primrose oil for the treatment of pre-menstrual syndrome.

Feverfew

Feverfew has been used traditionally for 'women's ailments' and inflammatory diseases. More recently it has been advocated as a treatment for headaches and migraine. A systematic review summarized all five double-blind, placebo-controlled randomized clinical trials in patients with headaches or migraine (Vogler *et al.*, 1998). Three of these studies suggested that feverfew is more efficacious than placebo in alleviating symptoms of this indication, while two trials showed no significant effects. The disagreement between the trials is likely to be due to the fact that parthenolides may not be, as previously thought, the (only) active constituent of feverfew. Clearly, more and better clinical trials are needed to evaluate the value of feverfew for headaches and migraine.

Garlic

For hypertension
Garlic has been advocated for centuries as a treatment of a variety of ailments. In particular, its cardioprotective properties such as lipid-lowering and blood pressure-lowering effects have been investi-

gated. The latter were summarized in a systematic review (Silagy and Neil, 1993) which included eight randomized clinical trials. The meta-analysis of these data suggests a small but statistically significant reduction in systolic and diastolic blood pressure.

For hypercholesterolaemia

The lipid-lowering properties of garlic have been assessed by a number of studies and meta-analyses (for example, Warshafsky *et al.*, 1993; Silagy and Neil, 1994; Berthold *et al.*, 1998). Most of the early trials suggested that garlic reduced total serum cholesterol levels. However, more recently a number of trials (Berthold *et al.*, 1998; Isaacsohn *et al.*, 1998) were published contradicting this notion. The reason for these differing results is as yet unclear. Thus, at present the efficacy of garlic for hypercholesterolaemia is uncertain. More data from rigorous trials or an update of the previous meta-analyses may provide the answers.

Ginger

Ginger has been in medicinal use since antiquity. Its antiemetic potential is supported by investigations in animals and healthy human volunteers. A systematic review of all six double-blind, placebo-controlled randomized clinical trials in human patients came to an overall positive conclusion (Ernst and Pittler, 1999a). With one exception, these studies suggest that ginger preparations are efficacious when compared with placebo in treating or preventing nausea or vomiting of various causes. Thus, the evidence for ginger as an antiemetic is tantalizing but unfortunately not ultimately compelling.

Ginkgo biloba

For cerebral insufficiency

Extracts from the leaves of the *Ginkgo biloba* or maidenhair tree are widely used for circulatory disorders such as peripheral vascular disease or cerebral insufficiency. A systematic review of *Ginkgo biloba* extract for the latter indication (Kleijnen and Knipschild, 1992) suggested beneficial effects when given for at least 4–6 weeks. A problem here is that cerebral insufficiency is an inadequately defined syndrome and not a universally accepted diagnosis.

For dementia

Intriguing evidence has emerged to suggest that *Ginkgo biloba* extract is also beneficial for dementia of either Alzheimer's or vascular type. The authors' systematic review included nine double-blind randomized clinical trials on the subject (Ernst and Pittler, 1999b). Some of these studies were of high methodological quality. The totality of the data suggest that the regular oral intake of *Ginkgo biloba* slows the loss of cognitive function in patients with dementia. Further studies are, however, required to define the optimal dose.

For tinnitus
Tinnitus – the perception of sound in the absence of external stimuli – affects about 6–14 per cent of the general population. Many treatments for this disturbing condition have been tried, but no gold standard exists. A recent systematic review (Ernst and Stevinson, 1999) included all five randomized clinical trials of *Ginkgo biloba* as a treatment for tinnitus. Overall, the results were favourable. Several caveats do, however, exist, and firm conclusions are therefore not possible.

For intermittent claudication
Treatment of intermittent claudication is usually conservative, and consists largely of regular physical exercise and/or oral drugs like pentoxifylline. A number of studies originating mainly from the German-speaking countries have assessed *Ginkgo biloba* for this condition. A meta-analysis (Pittler and Ernst, 1999a) of the available data suggests that *Ginkgo biloba* extract is superior to placebo in the symptomatic treatment of intermittent claudication. The size of the overall treatment effect is, however, modest.

Ginseng

A variety of different health claims are made for ginseng. A recent systematic review (Vogler *et al.*, 1999) found 16 double-blind randomized clinical trials. These trials relate to physical performance, psychomotor performance and cognitive function, immunomodulation, type 2 diabetes mellitus and herpes simplex type II infections. The evidence from this analysis is not compelling for any of these indications. The extremely widespread use of ginseng in the population renders more systematic investigations assessing its efficacy and safety a matter of urgency.

Hawthorn

Hawthorn has a similar pharmacological profile to digitalis, and it is frequently used on the European continent. It is effective beyond reasonable doubt in the early stages of congestive heart failure

(Weihmayr and Ernst, 1996). Mainstream medicine has, of course, a variety of highly effective drugs for treating congestive heart failure. In order to evaluate the relative value of hawthorn, trials comparing hawthorn preparations with commonly prescribed synthetic drugs are required. Too few such studies exist, at present, to make a reliable judgement.

Horse chestnut

Horse chestnut seed extract is widely used on the European continent as an oral and external treatment for varicose veins. The authors' systematic review (Pittler and Ernst, 1998b) included eight placebo-controlled randomized clinical trials on this topic. Collectively these data leave little doubt that horse chestnut seed extract is efficacious in reducing subjective symptoms and objective signs of chronic venous insufficiency. Five trials comparing horse chestnut seed extract with other active treatments were also reviewed. Their results imply that horse chestnut seed extract is as efficacious as various reference treatments.

Kava

Extracts of kava have been used for recreational and medicinal purposes throughout the South Pacific for hundreds of years. A recent systematic review and meta-analysis (Pittler and Ernst, 1999b) aimed to assess the evidence of kava extract as a symptomatic treatment for anxiety. Superiority of kava extract over placebo was suggested by all seven of the available trials. A meta-analysis suggested a significant difference in the reduction of the total score on the Hamilton Anxiety Scale in favour of kava extract. This systematic review therefore implied that kava is a herbal treatment for anxiety worthy of consideration.

Mistletoe

The evidence for the efficacy of mistletoe extract in the treatment of cancer has been summarized in a systematic review that included 11 controlled trials on the subject (Kleijnen and Knipschild, 1994). Although most trials yielded results that were in favour of mistletoe treatment, the study with the highest methodological quality did not corroborate these findings. Further well-performed and rigorous trials are therefore needed to determine the efficacy of mistletoe extract for this important indication.

Peppermint

Peppermint has been in traditional medicinal use for millennia. Relatively recently it has been tested as a treatment for irritable bowel syndrome. The authors' systematic review and meta-analysis of all randomized clinical trials included eight placebo-controlled studies (Pittler and Ernst, 1998c). The data collectively suggested that preparations of peppermint oil alleviate symptoms of irritable bowel syndrome significantly more than placebo. However, many trials are burdened with severe methodological flaws and thus preclude firm conclusions on the efficacy of peppermint oil for this indication.

Saw palmetto

Extracts of saw palmetto are widely used in Europe for symptoms associated with benign prostatic hypertrophy. In Germany, for instance, almost 90 per cent of all patients with this condition are treated with phytopharmaceutical agents, of which extracts of saw palmetto are the most popular preparations. Eighteen randomized trials assessing saw palmetto extract for benign prostatic hypertrophy were recently reviewed (Wilt *et al.*, 1998). The evidence suggested that the extract improves urologic symptoms and flow measures and is furthermore as efficacious as reference medications used for this condition.

St John's wort

St John's wort is a ubiquitous plant in the UK and other countries. It has been used for a long time for a range of indications including depressive disorders. In Germany, extracts of St John's wort are licensed for the treatment of anxiety and depressive and sleep disorders. A recent update paper (Stevinson and Ernst, 1999a) included six double-blind randomized trials of St John's wort extract for mild to moderate depression conducted since the publication of a previous meta-analysis (Linde *et al.*, 1996). Collectively, the results provided sound evidence demonstrating that St John's wort is superior to placebo in treating mild to moderate depression. The question of whether or not it is also effective for severe depression remains to be answered.

Table 6.1 Key data of systematic reviews and meta-analyses on the efficacy of herbal drugs*

Botanical (reference)	Indications	Methodology	Trials included	Average methodological quality	Main result	Comment
Aloe vera (Aloe barbadensis) (Vogler and Ernst, 1999)	Glucose-lowering, lipid-lowering, radiation injury, herpes, psoriasis, wound healing	SR	10	Poor	Some promising findings but no indication sufficiently documented	Promising indications are: diabetes, hyperlipidaemia, herpes, psoriasis
Artichoke (Cynara scolymus) (Pittler and Ernst, 1998a)	Hyperlipidaemia, dyspepsia	SR	1		More trials are needed to establish its efficacy for serum cholesterol reduction	A number of experimental studies support possible lipid-lowering effects
Feverfew (Tanacetum parthenium) (Vogler et al., 1998)	Headache/migraine prevention	SR	5	Good	Three trials were positive, and two were negative	Discrepancy of results could mean that parthenolides may not be, as previously assumed, the active principle
Ginger (Zingiber officinale) (Ernst and Pittler, 1999a)	Nausea/vomiting due to seasickness, morning sickness, chemotherapy, postoperative	SR	6	Good	Ginger seems more efficacious than placebo	Methodologically best study was negative
Ginkgo (Ginkgo biloba) (Ernst and Pittler, 1999b)	a. Dementia (Alzheimer's and vascular type)	SR	9	Good	Only one trial was negative	Dosage regimen varied by >100%
(Ernst and Stevinson, 1999)	b. Tinnitus	SR	5	Poor	Only one trial was negative	Methodologically best trial was positive
(Pittler and Ernst, 1999a)	c. Intermittent claudication	MA	8	Good to excellent	Overall positive result	Clinical relevance of effect is debatable

Table 6.1 (Continued)

Botanical (reference)	Indications	Methodology	Trials included	Average methodological quality	Main result	Comment
Ginseng (Vogler et al., 1999)	Various	SR	16	Poor	Evidence is compelling for none of the various indications	Physical performance and psychomotor performance/cognitive function are the best researched indications
Horse chestnut (Aesculus hippocastanum) (Pittler and Ernst, 1998b)	Chronic venous insufficiency	SR	8 vs. placebo, 5 vs. reference treatments	Good	Active treatment is more efficacious than placebo and equally efficacious as reference treatments	Both objective signs and subjective symptoms respond to treatment
Kava (Piper methysticum) (Pittler and Ernst, 1999b)	Anxiety	MA	7	Good	Superiority of kava extract over placebo is suggested by all trials	Reduction of the total score on the Hamilton Anxiety Scale
Peppermint (Mentha piperita) (Pittler and Ernst, 1998c)	Symptoms of irritable bowel syndrome (IBS)	MA	8	Poor	Although the MA is positive, peppermint oil has so far not been established beyond reasonable doubt for IBS	Only in one trial was IBS diagnosed according to accepted criteria
St John's wort (Hypericum perforatum) (Stevinson and Ernst, 1999a)	Depression	SR	6 published after earlier MA (Linde et al., 1996)	Excellent	Hypericum is more efficacious than placebo and may be as efficacious as synthetic antidepressants	This is an update of the evidence; one trial suggested that hypericum may also be efficacious for severe depression
Valerian (Valeriana officinalis) (Stevinson and Ernst, 1999b)	Insomnia	SR	9	Poor	Weak and contradictory evidence prevents firm conclusions	Great inconsistency between trials concerning patients, design and procedures

Table is confined to recent research done by the authors. Only double-blind randomized controlled trials have been included except for Vogler and Ernst (1999) and Ernst and Stevinson (1999). SR, systematic review; MA, meta-analysis.

Valerian

Valerian is in frequent use for promoting sleep. In many countries, valerian extracts are marketed as an over-the-counter product for this purpose with considerable success. Perhaps surprisingly, the evidence for its efficacy was almost entirely anecdotal until recently. A systematic review located nine double-blind randomized clinical trials on the subject (Stevinson and Ernst, 1999b). Great inconsistencies in these trials in terms of patients treated, experimental design and other methodological details prevent firm conclusions regarding the efficacy of valerian as a treatment for insomnia. *Vis-à-vis* its widespread use, definitive randomized clinical trials are now urgently needed.

Comment

This brief overview of systematic reviews demonstrates that the findings, as expected, vary according to plant extract and indication. In many cases the overall result is not as compelling as anticipated. The reasons for this are diverse. The most prevalent ones are the relative paucity of randomized clinical trials available for a systematic review of their efficacy, and the numerous methodological flaws in trials of herbal treatments. Yet in some cases the evidence is sound and convincing.

Although systematic reviews represent the highest level of scientific evidence, they are clearly not without drawbacks. In fact, their shortcomings are numerous. If, for instance, flawed randomized clinical trials are evaluated, the results of a systematic review are similarly distorted. However, this does not necessarily affect the conclusions of a systematic review. One of the strengths of systematic reviews is to identify flawed trials (for example, Pittler and Ernst, 1998c) and point out their limitations. This information can then be used constructively to work towards filling important gaps in the present knowledge.

Other problems associated with systematic reviews and meta-analyses include publication bias. Negative trials tend to remain unpublished both in mainstream and complementary medicine (Easterbrook *et al.*, 1991; Ernst and Pittler, 1997), and thus the published evidence might become biased towards a false positive overall conclusion. In systematic reviews an attempt should be made to minimize this drawback by inviting experts on a particular subject, as well as manufacturers, to contribute unpublished material. However, there is no guarantee that they will comply and therefore it is never entirely certain whether all existing evidence has been included.

It has been shown that the English language medical literature tends to be biased towards positive results, and negative trials tend to emerge in journals publishing in other languages (Egger *et al.*, 1997). It is therefore important not to restrict systematic reviews to the English language literature. In herbal medicine this is of particular relevance since, for historical reasons, a lot of the data are published in German or French. As far as the authors' systematic reviews are concerned, they made a point of including languages other than English.

In herbal medicine there are further problems which relate to the (lack of) standardization of extracts. If one preparation of a given herb is shown to be effective, this does not necessarily mean that another preparation of the same herb is similarly effective. If, subsequently, all trials of different preparations of one herb are systematically reviewed or meta-analysed, there is a considerable risk of distortion. Except for insisting that all herbal preparations be adequately standardized, there is no easy way around this problem. A review of studies with inadequately standardized preparations may produce a false negative overall result. It is, however, unlikely that it will produce a false positive finding. In essence, at least with respect to extract quality, positive systematic reviews are reliable while negative ones provide a good reason for conducting sub-analyses according to extract specificity.

It is concluded that systematic reviews are a useful, albeit not infallible, approach to assess the efficacy of herbal medicines. Using this approach, compelling positive results for some herbal remedies have been found, while for other plant extracts more work needs to be done to determine their efficacy.

References

Berthold, H. K., Sudhop, T. and von Bergamann, K. (1998). Effect of a garlic oil preparation on serum lipoproteins and cholesterol metabolism: a randomized controlled trial. *JAMA*, **279**, 1900–02.

Budeiri, D., Li Wan Po, A. and Dornan, J. C. (1996). Is evening primrose oil of value in the treatment of pre-menstrual syndrome? *Contr. Clin. Trials*, **17**, 60–68.

Crombie, I. K. and McQuay, H. J. (1998). The systematic review: a good guide rather than a guarantee. *Pain*, **76**, 1–2.

Easterbrook, P. J., Berlin, J. A., Gopalan, R. and Matthews, D. R. (1991). Publication bias in clinical research. *Lancet*, **337**, 867–72.

Egger, M., Zellweger-Zähner, T., Schneider, M. *et al.* (1997). Language bias in randomised controlled trials published in English and German. *Lancet,* **350**, 326–9.

Eisenberg, D., David, R. B., Ettner, S. L. *et al.* (1998).Trends in alternative medicine use in the United States, 1990–1997. *JAMA,* **280**, 1569–75.

Ernst, E. and Pittler, M. H. (1997). Alternative therapy bias. *Nature,* **385**, 480.

Ernst, E. and Pittler, M. H. (1999a). Ginger for nausea and vomiting. A systematic review. *Br. J. Anaesth.* (in press).

Ernst, E. and Pittler, M. H. (1999b). *Ginkgo biloba* for dementia: a systematic review of double-blind placebo-controlled trials. *Clin. Drug Invest.,* **17**, 301–8.

Ernst, E. and Stevinson, C. (1999). *Ginkgo biloba* for tinnitus: a review. *Clin. Otolaryngol.,* **24**, 164–7.

Isaacsohn, J. L., Moser, M., Stein, E. A. *et al.* (1998). Garlic powder and plasma lipids and lipoproteins. *Arch. Intern. Med.,* **158**, 1189–94.

Kleijnen, J. and Knipschild, P. (1992). *Ginkgo biloba* for cerebral insufficiency. *Br. J. Clin. Pharmacol.,* **34**, 352–8.

Kleijnen, J. and Knipschild, P. (1994). Mistletoe treatment for cancer. Review of controlled trials in humans. *Phytomedicine,* **1**, 255–60.

Linde, K., Ramirez, G., Mulrow, C. D. *et al.* (1996). St John's wort for depression – an overview and meta-analysis of randomised clinical trials. *Br. Med. J.,* **313**, 253–8.

Melchart, D., Linde, K., Fischer, P. and Kaesmayr, J. (1999). Echinacea for the prevention and treatment of the common cold (Cochrane review). *The Cochrane Library,* Issue 1. Update Software.

Pittler, M. H. and Ernst, E. (1998a). Artichoke leaf extract for serum cholesterol reduction. *Perfusion,* **11**, 338–40.

Pittler, M. H. and Ernst, E. (1998b). Horse-chestnut seed extract for chronic venous insufficiency: A criteria-based systematic review. *Arch. Dermatol.,* **134**, 1356–60.

Pittler, M. H. and Ernst, E. (1998c). Peppermint oil for irritable bowel syndrome: a critical review and meta-analysis. *Am. J. Gastroenterol.,* **93**, 1131–5.

Pittler, M. H. and Ernst, E. (1999a) *Ginkgo biloba* extract for the treatment of intermittent claudication. A meta-analysis *Am. J. Med.* (in press).

Pittler, M. H. and Ernst E. (1999b) Kava as a treatment for anxiety. A systematic review and meta-analysis *J. Clin. Psychopharmacol.* (in press).

Silagy, C. A. and Neil, A. W. (1993). A meta-analysis of the effect of garlic on blood pressure. *J. Hypertension,* **12**, 463–8.

Silagy, C. A. and Neil, A. W. (1994). Garlic as a lipid-lowering agent – a meta-analysis. *J. R. Coll. Phys. Lond.,* **28**, 2–8.

Stevinson, C. and Ernst. E. (1999a). Hypericum for depression: an update of the clinical evidence. *Eur. Neuropsychopharmacol.* (in press).

Stevinson, C. and Ernst, E. (1999b) Valerian for insomnia? A systematic review. (submitted).

Vogler, B. K. and Ernst, E. (1999). Aloe vera: a systematic review of its clinical effectiveness. *Br. J. Gen. Pract.* (in press).

Vogler, B. K., Pittler, M. H. and Ernst, E. (1998). Feverfew as a preventive treatment for migraine: a systematic review. *Cephalalgia,* **18**, 704–8.

Vogler, B. K., Pittler, M. H. and Ernst, E. (1999) The efficacy of ginseng. A systematic review of randomized clinical trials. *Eur. J. Clin. Pharmacol.* (in press).
Warshafsky, S., Kamer, R. S. and Sivak, S. L. (1993). Effect of garlic on total serum cholesterol: a meta-analysis. *Ann. Int. Med.*, **119**, 599–605.
Weihmayr, Th. and Ernst, E. (1996). Die Therapeutische Wirksamkeit von Crataegus. *Fortschr. Med.*, **114**, 27–9.
Wilt, T. J., Ishani, A., Stark, G. *et al.* (1998). Saw palmetto extracts for treatment of benign prostatic hyperplasia. *JAMA*, **280**, 1604–9.

7

Safety issues in phytotherapy

S. B. A. Halkes

Introduction

In the twentieth century, following the advances in biological and medical sciences and organic chemistry that resulted in the introduction of powerful synthetic drugs, the use of medicinal plant preparations (phytomedicines) in modern medicine strongly declined. However, currently a revival of interest in phytomedicines is to be observed. Many patients nowadays tend to abandon synthetic drugs and turn to herbal remedies for the treatment of their illnesses. The main reason for this development seems to be the general belief that natural products are harmless or at least have fewer side effects than regular drugs. To accommodate the needs of consumers, pharmaceutical industries have started marketing an increasing amount of (new) phytomedicines. Consequently, the expenditure on phytomedicines has become substantial over the last few years and is still growing rapidly (Grünwald, 1995; Brevoort, 1996; Blumenthal and Tyler, 1997).

As a result of the growing popularity of phytomedicines, the need for the assessment of quality, safety and efficacy of these products is increasingly felt. In particular, the evaluation of safety aspects should have priority since the above-mentioned assumption that phytomedicines only have beneficial effects has proven to be incorrect. Although the number of side effects associated with the use of phytomedicines represents only a small proportion of the total amount of adverse drug reactions in the WHO database (Barnes, 1998), reports on toxic effects of or adverse reactions to herbal preparations have regularly been published over the past years (for example, Fox *et al.*, 1978; Galizia, 1983; Kumana *et al.*, 1983; Roulet *et al.*, 1989; De Smet *et al.*, 1990; Vale, 1998).

Toxicity related to the use of phytomedicines may have multiple causes, but in general two categories can be distinguished (Table 7.1). The first category can be designated as extrinsic or non-plant-associated; toxic effects or adverse reactions occurring because of accidental or deliberate contamination or substitution of the plant material described on the label. The second category is more intrinsic or plant-associated in nature. In this category, the plant material itself, as the active ingredient in the herbal medicinal product, produces the health risks.

Table 7.1 Causative factors involved in the occurrence of adverse drug reactions to herbal medicinal products

Extrinsic or non-plant-associated causes; health risks related to contamination, substitution or adulteration of the plant material

1. Contamination:
   - Heavy metals (lead, mercury, cadmium, etc.)
   - Pesticides and/or herbicides
   - Micro-organisms (bacteria, including *E. coli* and Salmonella, yeasts, moulds)
   - Microbial toxins (aflatoxins, lipopolysaccharides)
   - Radioactivity
   - Fumigants
2. Substitution:
   - Animal substances (enzymes, hormones, organ extracts, etc.)
   - Synthetic drugs (corticosteroids, anti-inflammatory agents, etc.)
3. Adulteration:
   - Accidental or deliberate substitution of the original plant material by other plant species

Intrinsic or plant-associated causes; health risks related to the medicinal herb itself, as active ingredient in the phytomedicine

1. Ignored toxicity of a plant(constituent) present in the product
2. Use of plants, either as raw material or in processed form, of which at present no or insufficient data regarding safety are available
3. Use of highly concentrated or specifically processed extracts
4. Use of plants containing constituents that are known to affect bioavailability and/or pharmacokinetics of other compounds or drugs

The objective of this chapter is to give a brief overview of the points to consider with regard to both types of toxicity. In addition, as far as they are related to safety issues, experiences acquired in a recent survey of herbal medicinal products available on the Dutch market and initial evaluation of some product dossiers (Commissie Toetsing Fytotherapeutica, 1999) will be presented.

Adverse drug reactions associated with contamination or substitution of the plant material

A critical evaluation of the available reports in which adverse drug reactions to phytomedicines have been described shows that in many cases toxicity was due to contamination or substitution of the plant material. The risks associated with the use of such contaminated or adulterated herbal products have been reviewed extensively by De Smet (1992a). Therefore, this aspect of herbal safety will only be briefly commented upon here.

. Contaminants most likely to be found in crude medicinal herbs include heavy metals (lead, mercury, cadmium), pesticides and/or herbicides, micro-organisms, microbial toxins (lipopolysaccharides as well as aflatoxins) and radioactive isotopes. It is evident that the presence of such contaminants is inherent to the production process of vegetal materials and cannot be excluded completely. However, contamination may be significantly reduced when cultivation and harvesting are carried out in accordance with good agricultural practice guidelines, such as those formulated by the European organization of medicinal plant producers (Europam, 1998). Furthermore, the risks of contamination highlight the need for adequate control of the pharmaceutical quality of the finished products derived from medicinal plants. In this respect, the requirements with regard to the quality control of phytomedicines that must be fulfilled before a marketing authorization is granted for the European Community (European Commission, 1998a) are certainly legitimate.

Besides contamination, adulteration of the original plant material or substitution with synthetic or animal substances is regularly observed in herbal medicinal products. This is often the result of ignorance or incompetence, but cases of deliberate substitution with cheaper or more common plant species and conventional drugs have been described. Another potential cause of adulteration is the botanical nomenclature. The extensive use of vernacular names in particular may lead to confusion over the identity of particular herbs used in a phytomedicine.

Since the use of various chromatographic techniques such as thin-layer chromatography (TLC), high-performance liquid chromatography (HPLC), etc., have made it possible to unambiguously identify the ingredients in a phytomedicine, good-quality assurance can also effectively prevent the detrimental effects that these adulterated or substituted preparations may inflict on general health. In addition, to counteract confusion over terminology, it is important to use the binomial designation for plants throughout all product labelling.

Plant-associated adverse drug reactions

A considerable number of plants, especially herbs used in foods and traditional medicinal plants, have a well-documented history of safe use. For these plants, no reports on the occurrence of serious side effects, irrespective of the dosage, have been published, and therefore it is not likely that they cause adverse drug reactions. Many of these 'safe' herbs are included in lists like that of the German Kommission E (Blumenthal *et al.*, 1998) or the American Herbal Products Association (where they are defined as Class 1 herbs; herbs that can be consumed safely when used appropriately – McGuffin *et al.*, 1997). In general, it can be assumed that phytomedicines prepared from this group of plants do not pose serious health risks and therefore can be exempt from specific restrictive regulatory actions and sold freely.

Other plants and herbal medicinal products may well have health risks, and their safety cannot be guaranteed unless additional requirements are met. In particular, evidence should be supplied to prove the preparation is innocuous before a marketing authorization is granted. The next sections will be devoted to the specific problems that these products may pose, and the measures required to ensure their safe use.

Definition of the safety problems involved in the use of herbal medicinal products

In the course of determining the health risks related to the use of phytomedicines and the problems that are involved in this respect, it may be useful to categorize herbal medicinal products according to the plants from which they are derived and the way in which they are processed. The groups are as follows:

1. Phytomedicines containing known toxic plant material or extracts thereof
2. Phytomedicines containing plants, either as raw material or in processed form, of which at present no or insufficient scientific data regarding their safety are available
3. Phytomedicines containing extracts that have, in addition to

the currently used extraction procedures, been subjected to specific manufacturing processes – e.g. highly concentrated, enriched or partially purified extracts

4. Phytomedicines containing plants or plant constituents that are known to affect the bioavailability and/or pharmacokinetics of other compounds or drugs.

The specific risks related to the use of each of these herbal medicinal products will be discussed in the following paragraphs.

Phytomedicines with toxic ingredients

It has long been recognized that certain plants or plant constituents are toxic and that their use may be hazardous and can cause health risks (Röder, 1982; Roth *et al.*, 1984; De Smet, 1992b). The application of these herbs as phytomedicines is in general obsolete and should be discouraged. This category includes plants such as *Aconitum napellus*, *Rubia tinctorum*, *Digitalis* species, *Croton tiglium* (fatty oil from the seeds) and *Ricinus communis*. The use of these plants is restricted by statutory regulation in many countries.

Despite the legislatory exclusion of some notorious toxic plant species, the use of other potentially harmful herbs still persists, as may be concluded from a recent survey in The Netherlands (Commissie Toetsing Fytotherapeutica, 1999) and previous observations on the German phytomedicine market (Thesen, 1988). For obvious reasons, the availability of such potentially noxious plants, and galenic preparations thereof, is a cause for concern.

Phytomedicines containing herbal ingredients for which insufficient safety data are available

Although prescribers and consumers of phytomedicines will be able to recognize major adverse drug reactions such as dermatological reactions, nausea and disturbances of the gastrointestinal tract, other more subtle symptoms of toxicity may easily be missed. Consequently, in many cases it has proved difficult to demonstrate a clear association between the occurrence of adverse effects and the use of a particular herb. For this reason, only a small number of plants are characterized as toxic and are treated as such. However, there are many other herbs, including perhaps even those generally considered safe, which may pose potential harmful effects. This is particularly true in the case of plants or herbal products for which no scientific or clinical data are available with respect to carcinogenic, mutagenic or teratogenic activities and long-term use. Since noxious effects cannot be excluded, these plants and products must be considered as potentially toxic.

Phytomedicines containing specifically processed extracts
In recent years an increasing number of phytomedicines have been
marketed that contain specifically processed extracts, e.g. highly
concentrated, enriched or partially purified extracts. The profile of
constituents present in such preparations may differ substantially
from ordinary extracts (percolates, macerates, tinctures, etc.), both in
qualitative and quantitative aspects. For example, Wagner *et al.*
(1989) found significant differences in the TLC and HPLC
characteristics of a selectively enriched *ginkgo* extract used in
several commercial preparations, as compared to normal methanolic
or ethanolic extracts. Accordingly, the total concentration of
terpenoids in *Ginkgo biloba* leaf extracts and phytopharmaceuticals
was found to vary greatly (Van Beek *et al.*, 1991). Due to these
deviations in composition, it is unlikely that toxicity data obtained
with trivial extracts can provide an accurate and reliable insight into
the actual dangers of preparations containing specifically processed
extracts. Therefore, in the safety assessment of such phytomedicines
it is not justifiable to refer to toxicological data from other
preparations.

*Phytomedicines with plants or plant constituents affecting
bioavailability and/or pharmacokinetics*
Several plants or plant constituents are renowned for their ability to
affect the bioavailability and pharmacokinetics of co-administered
drugs. In particular, the major alkaloid component in *Piper* species,
piperine, can be mentioned in this respect. Piperine has been reported
to increase serum concentrations of drugs such as the bronchodilator
theophylline and the beta-blocker propranolol (Bano *et al.*, 1991) and
also the plant constituent curcumin (Shoba *et al.*, 1998) after oral
administration in laboratory animals and humans. This enhancement
of systemic availability by piperine is probably related to the
inhibition of glucuronidation in the liver and the small intestine (Atal
et al., 1985; Singh *et al.*, 1986). Other plant constituents that may
influence the biopharmaceutical parameters of a phytomedicine
include saponins and essential oil constituents, the former being able
to increase the water solubility of apolar compounds (Nakayama *et
al.*, 1986; Schöpke and Bartlakowski, 1997) and the latter improving
percutaneous absorption (Hori *et al*, 1991; Williams and Barry, 1991).
   Plants containing this type of constituent may have distinct safety
problems. The ability of such compounds to influence the
bioavailability and/or pharmacokinetics of additional ingredients,
particularly when they are used in complex or combined
preparations, may significantly alter the toxicological profile of
these products. Ayurvedic preparations should be considered in this

respect, since extracts of *Piper* species are part of most formulations used in this Indian traditional medical system.

Requirements for the safe use of phytomedicines

Having described in broad outline the difficulties that might be encountered in relation to the safety of medicinal herbs, the next step is to consider in more detail some approaches to dealing with these problems. The specific requirements needed for the safe use of herbal medicinal products containing potentially toxic plants or plant constituents will be covered in a separate paragraph. Although the other problems highlighted above are diverse, the measures to be taken to control the health risks posed in general demand the same approach; thorough research into the toxicological potential of the extracts or products in question. Therefore, this aspect will also be touched upon below.

Minimizing the risks associated with the use of toxic botanicals

Herbal medicinal products containing potentially toxic plants or plant constituents may at present be a cause for concern unless clear restrictions are issued for their use. In this respect, it would first be prudent to limit the use of potentially toxic herbs to those cases in which the established or putative beneficial effects of the plant in question clearly outweigh the health risks; for example, *Valeriana officinalis*, which contains valepotriates. These constituents, as well as their metabolites, have been shown to possess *in vitro* cytotoxic and mutagenic activity, probably attributable to their alkylating properties (Bos *et al.*, 1997). However, there is reasonable doubt as to whether the toxic effects of valepotriates are of relevance in humans, since they are absent or only present in minute quantities in commercial preparations (Van Meer *et al.*, 1977) and little is resorbed from the intestinal tract in unchanged form (Wagner and Jurcic, 1980). In conjunction with the beneficial potential of valerian preparations in the treatment of sleep disorders (European Scientific Co-operative on Phytotherapy, 1997), it can be concluded that the risk–benefit analysis has an advantageous outcome for this plant.

Secondly, even though a risk–benefit analysis yields positive results, it may be desirable to restrict the content of toxic constituents to the lowest possible levels. In this regard it is important to distinguish between toxic constituents that do not contribute to the biological and/or medicinal properties of the herb, and pharmacologically active compounds which may, in higher doses, provide health risks.

In the case of plants containing constituents which have only been implicated in the production of toxic effects or adverse reactions, without being involved in the beneficial effects, it is important to reduce the concentration of these compounds to the absolute minimum. This can be achieved not only by careful selection of chemical races (plant parts used in a herbal preparation) and growing or harvesting conditions of the plant material, but also by choosing selective extraction procedures and/or additional purification steps. The former factors have been found significantly to influence the levels of toxins, as is exemplified by reference to the following literature data:

- The content of the phenylpropane derivative β-asarone, which showed carcinogenic activity in several *in vivo* studies, is dependent on the number of chromosomes in *Acorus calamus*; commercial products prepared from an American diploid variety contain no traceable amounts of β-asarone whereas those of European (triploid) and Indian (tetraploid) varieties yielded low and high concentrations respectively of this compound (Stahl and Keller, 1981).
- Roots of *Symphytum asperum* have higher levels of alkaloids in comparison to the aerial parts (Roitman, 1981). Likewise, ginkgolic acids are detectable in both the leaves and seed covers of *Ginkgo biloba*, but relative concentrations in the leaves are so low that allergic responses, especially dermatitis, can be excluded (Wagner *et al.*, 1989).
- The pyrrolizidine alkaloid content in the leaves of different *Senecio* species varied widely depending on the time of year or developmental stage at which the plant was collected (Johnson *et al.*, 1985). Similar results were obtained with regard to the seasonal variation in the amounts of the neurotoxin 4-O-methylpyridoxine in *Ginkgo biloba* leaves and seeds (Arenz *et al.*, 1996).
- The concentration of alkaloids in *Senecio* species was found to be affected by the area in which the plants are collected (Johnson *et al.*, 1985).

When the above-mentioned factors do not or only inadequately apply, consideration should be given to lowering the content of toxic constituents in herbal preparations through the selective elimination of these compounds. Sometimes it is possible to prevent the extraction of unwanted constituents simply by using the correct solvent system. In other instances, however, this will prove to be inadequate, and more specific separation or purification procedures are needed in order to achieve the desired result. For example, the basic characteristic of alkaloids can in general be used to remove them from extracts. The amine function allows the possibility of transferring these constituents from aqueous solutions to apolar solvents under alkaline conditions, and alkaloids can again be extracted from the lipophilic phase in acidified water (Steinegger and Hänsel, 1988).

However, complete reduction of the levels of a potentially toxic component is not always possible in order to minimize the health risks associated with the use of a herbal preparation. This is particularly true when a phytomedicine contains constituents that are both pharmacologically active and detrimental, depending on the dosage; removal of these constituents will also render the product ineffective. In such cases it may be useful to specify limits for the components in question, as is done in the European Pharmacopoeia for the content of hydroxyanthracene derivatives in standardized *aloe* dry extracts (*European Pharmacopoeia*, 1989).

Finally, from the point of view of safety, the application of a use restriction for potentially noxious plants or plant preparations might be appropriate. For instance, to prevent hepatic damage (veno-occlusive disease) due to long-term exposure to pyrrolizidine-containing plants such as *Symphytum* and *Petasites* species, it may be appropriate to limit the use of such herbs to external use only and to warn against prolonged use or application to open wounds (McGuffin *et al.*, 1997). Likewise, it seems advisable to include a caution regarding hypersensitivity and allergic reactions in the product labelling of phytomedicines containing plants from the Asteraceae (= Compositae) family (Wichtl, 1994).

The necessity for toxicological evaluation of herbal medicinal products

Where insufficient data are available or reasonable doubt exists as to whether or not a specific phytomedicine can be used safely (e.g. in the case of phytomedicines described previously), complementary evidence should be supplied to prove that such a preparation is innocuous. In this regard, it seems preferable to consider phytomedicines as regular medicines. Thus, like all new drugs that are being filed for marketing authorization, herbal medicinal products should satisfy the requirements for the acceptance of safe use as laid down by, for example, the European Community (European Commission, 1998b). Usually this will require thorough research into the extracts or products in question. Knowledge about the acute, sub-acute and chronic toxicity, any potentially harmful effects on reproduction including embryo/foetal and perinatal toxicity, mutagenic and carcinogenic activity, tolerance and pharmacokinetic parameters, etc., should be established to minimize the health risks (Table 7.2).

Table 7.2 Toxicological studies generally required for the assessment of drug safety (compiled from Hodgson, 1987, and European Commission, 1998a)

Single dose toxicity tests:
- Assessment of acute toxic potential (general behavioural and histopathological alterations, etc.)
- Establishing dose–effect relationships
- Lethal dose finding (LD_{50} test)

Repeated dose toxicity tests:
- Evaluation of sub-acute or chronic toxicity (behavioural and histopathological changes, aberrations in growth, haematological and biochemical parameters, etc.)
- Determination of the oncogenic properties (tumour incidence)

Assays for reproductive toxicity:
- Assessment of potential detrimental effects on fertility and general reproductive performances (changes in spermatogenesis and/or ovulatory cycle, pre- and post-implantation deaths, duration of gestation, litter size and condition of progeny, etc.)
- Determination of teratogenic activity (internal and external malformations in the embryo and/or foetus)
- Establishing effects in late pregnancy and lactation (alterations in growth performance)

Mutagenicity and carcinogenicity tests:
- Evaluation of possible effects on genetic material (Ames test, assay for sister chromatid exchange, etc.)

Special toxicity tests:
- Assessment of specific toxic effects such as neurotoxicity, immunotoxicity, etc.

Tolerance studies:
- Establishing the tolerability of bodily tissues which may come in contact with the drug directly after administration

Clinical trials and post-marketing surveillance studies:
- Evaluation of the adverse drug reactions occurring in the strict settings of a clinical trial and in real-life situations
- Determination of possible interactions with other drugs (of synthetic or natural origin)

Only few exceptions can be made to the general rule that herbal medicinal products should be scrupulously investigated for toxic effects. For instance, when it can be demonstrated that the extract manufactured as a phytomedicine is identical (equivalent) to extracts previously tested, information may be extracted from bibliographic data regarding the toxicity of the latter. Furthermore, the requirement for a herbal medicinal product to comply with detailed toxicological studies diminishes when it can be shown that its consumption does not pose real health threats. Such proof of safety can be provided by post-marketing surveillance studies of an already marketed phytomedicine.

Outcomes of a recent survey of herbal products in The Netherlands

With the exception of a few registered phytomedicines, herbal products sold in The Netherlands do not carry any medical claims or specific indications. They are therefore not considered as drugs under Dutch legislation, and are not examined as such by the Medicines Evaluation Board. As a consequence, herb-containing preparations are not required to fulfil the strict rules set for drugs and can be marketed with only few restrictions as food supplements and health-promoting agents. In order to monitor the quality, safety and efficacy of these herbal products more adequately, the Commissie Toetsing Fytotherapeutica (CTF; Committee for the Assessment of Phytomedicines) was founded in 1990 by private law arrangement on the initiative of the NVF (Dutch Association for Phytotherapy) and NEHOMA (Dutch Association for Manufacturers and Importers of Homoeopathics and Phytomedicines). To reach the goal of a self-regulating system for the control of herbal products, the CTF started in 1997 with a survey of such preparations available on the Dutch market and an initial dossier-evaluation of some of those products (Commissie Toetsing Fytotherapeutica, 1999). The results of this study, as far as they relate to safety aspects, are described below. The topics raised in this respect may serve to illustrate the need for adequate quality control and toxicological evaluation of herbal products as previously discussed in this chapter.

Data acquisition for the survey proceeded through direct mailing to the industry, with the request to list their herbal products. Moreover, advertisements in health periodicals, free local papers, etc. were screened. In this way, information on 1505 products containing plant material was collected. The majority of these herbal preparations could be classified as monopreparations (474 products, containing only one single plant component), complex preparations (540 products, containing material of more than one plant species), and combined preparations (191 products, containing single chemical entities as active ingredients, along with herbal components). The remaining herbal products could not be categorized due to inadequate data (Figure 7.1a).

(a) Herbal products

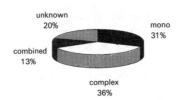

unknown
20%

mono
31%

combined
13%

complex
36%

(b) Total number of plants   (c) Most frequently used plants

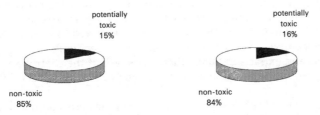

potentially
toxic
15%

potentially
toxic
16%

non-toxic
85%

non-toxic
84%

Figure 7.1 Results of a recent survey of herbal products in The Netherlands (Commissie Toetsing Fytotherapeutica, 1999)

Most of the herbal products were presented as true pharmaceuticals in which powdered plant materials or extracts were formulated into tablets, capsules, liquids or topical preparations. Other preparations with herbal ingredients were found to be less well-defined, and consisted of health-promoting products such as herbal teas, vitamin or food supplements, essential oils, cosmetics, etc.

The survey activities yielded a total of 798 specific plant species that were used in herbal products. Approximately 10–15 per cent of these plants could be identified as potentially noxious or even plainly toxic, e. g. several *Aconitum* species and also *Petasites* and *Symphytum* species (Figure 7.1b). In the group of the 25 most frequently used plants, four were found to have caused considerable controversy in the literature as to whether or not they constitute health risks (Figure 7.1c). These plants included *Viscum album*, *Arnica montana*, *Juniperus communis* and *Ruta graveolens*. The first two in particular should be regarded with caution. *Viscum album* is in the list of the top 10 plants implicated in adverse drug reaction reports as compiled by the WHO Collaborating Centre for International Drug Monitoring (Barnes, 1998), and *Arnica montana* ranks Class 3 (to be used only under the supervision of an expert qualified in the appropriate use of this substance) for internal use in the safety list of the American Herbal Products Association (McGuffin *et al.*, 1997).

The quality, safety, and efficacy of eight herbal preparations marketed in The Netherlands were assessed in more detail. For this purpose, product dossiers were obtained from the manufacturers. The preparations relevant to these dossiers contained extracts of the following plants or plant parts as active ingredients: *Chelidonium majus, Echinacea purpurea, Glycyrrhiza glabra, Hypericum perforatum, Matricaria recutita, Melissa officinalis, Panax ginseng,* and *Valeriana officinalis.*

In general, only very limited information concerning the origin of the plant material was presented in the dossiers; particulars with regard to the growing and harvesting conditions of the herbs were described in only three dossiers (Table 7.3). Other aspects of the quality assurance of the products were well substantiated. Comprehensive information regarding the identification of plant material and extracts obtained thereof, as well as the control for the presence of possible contaminants, was supplied in all dossiers (Table 7.3).

In the majority of dossiers, the safe use of the herbal products was poorly documented. In four dossiers, such proof of safety was based solely upon literature data, whereas for one product an additional tentative study into the tolerability of the product and the occurrence of adverse drug reactions was performed. A firm scientific basis for their safe use was provided for just three products. These were extensively tested for *in vitro* and *in vivo* toxicity, for acute and chronic toxicity, mutagenicity, carcinogenicity and teratogenic or foetotoxic activity. These products were also screened for adverse drug effects, both in the strictly controlled settings of clinical trials and in post-marketing surveillance studies (Table 7.3).

Conclusion

The total number of plant species in the world may well exceed half a million. Medicinal properties have been attributed to a considerable percentage of these plants and they are used in a multitude of preparations, including phytomedicines, health-promoting products and dietary supplements or food additives. The consumer should be provided with reliable and safe phytomedicines, and for this reason it is essential to assess the health risks involved in the use of these products. This does not mean that it should be assumed that all herbal products are harmless, as some advocates of natural remedies would have it. Neither should the use of botanicals be unconditionally rejected as dangerous nonsense, as may be done by biased

Table 7.3 Pharmaceutical and toxicological analysis of eight herbal products marketed in The Netherlands (Commissie Toetsing Fytotherapeutica, 1999)

Phytomedicine	1[1]	2	3	4	5	6	7	8
Quality control of plant material:								
Origin specified	?	?	n	n	n	y	y	y
GAP-guidelines applied	n	?				y	y	y
Inspection for identity	y	y	y	y	n	y	y	y
Inspection for contamination	y	y	y	y	y	y	y	y
• Heavy metals	+	+	?	0	0	+	+	+
• Pesticides and/or herbicides	+	+	+	+	+	+	+	+
• Micro-organisms	x	x	x	+	0	0	0	+
• Aflatoxins	+	+	+	+	+	+	+	+
Quality control of finished product:								
Inspection for identity	y	n	y	y	y	y	y	y
• Thin-layer chromatography	+		+	+	+	+	+	+
• High-performance liquid chromatography	+		0	0	0	+	+	0
• Other	0		0	0	+	0	0	0
Inspection for contamination	y	n	y	y	y	y	y	y
• Micro-organisms	+		+	+	0	+	+	+
Safety assessment of the finished product:								
Based on literature data	y	y	y	y	y	y	y	y
Based on toxicological studies	y	n	n	n	n	y	y	y
• *In vitro* tests	n					y	y	y
• *In vivo* tests	n					y	y	y
• Clinical studies	y					y	y	y
Tolerance study	y					n	n	y
Adverse effects in clinical trials	n					y	y	y
Adverse effects in post-marketing surveillance studies	n					y	y	y

The extract used to manufacture the finished product was controlled for identity and contaminations.
[1]: numbers depicted encode for the eight products evaluated
?: insufficient data in the dossier
y: data available in the dossier
n: no data available in the dossier
+: in accordance with requirements set in the European Pharmacopoeia, legislation, etc.
0: not tested
x: not in accordance with requirements set in the European Pharmacopoeia, legislation, etc.

critics. In considering the different safety aspects of herbal medicinal products, an objective scientific attitude should be adopted.

The issues to be addressed with respect to the safety assessment of herbal medicinal products have been discussed in this chapter. Like conventional drugs, these kinds of products should be adequately controlled for pharmaceutical quality in order to prevent contamination, substitution or adulteration. Furthermore, the application of known toxic plants should be restricted and limited to those instances in which the established or putative beneficial effects of the plant clearly outweigh the health risks. Even then, all possible measures should be taken to reduce the concentration of toxic compounds to the absolute minimum.

Where available data are unsatisfactory, or in case of reasonable doubt as to the safe use of a phytomedicine, complementary evidence in the form of toxicological studies should be supplied to prove that the preparation is innocuous.

A few other points may be worth considering to safeguard the consumer against potential health risks. For instance, attention should be drawn to the fact that some users may be more susceptible to adverse drug reactions than others. In particular, long-term users, consumers of large amounts of phytomedicines or people who use many different medicinal products may be prone to side effects. Pregnant or nursing women, babies, the elderly, sick and malnourished or undernourished are also at higher risk (Huxtable, 1990). It is essential that these users are made aware of the hazards and that they are properly informed. Since most herbal medicinal products are non-prescription drugs, it is of the utmost importance that the manufacturer provides comprehensible cautionery leaflets (De Smet, 1992a). In this respect, it is also important that patients notify their general practitioner if they are taking phytomedicines concurrently with conventional drugs – especially with cardiac, diuretic, sedative, hypotensive or other properties, since plant products with similar activities may enhance their effects (Newall *et al.*, 1996).

Acknowledgement

The author thanks all members of the Commissie Toetsing Fytotherapeutica for their respective contributions to the described work. The assistance of Ms S. F. des Tombe in the survey activities and in the preparation of this manuscript is gratefully acknowledged. Doctors J. H. van Meer and S. Pos are thanked for helpful discussion.

References

Arenz, A., Klein, M., Fiehe, K. *et al.* (1996). Occurrence of neurotoxic 4-O-methylpyridoxine in *Ginkgo biloba* leaves, ginkgo medications and Japanese ginkgo food. *Planta Med.*, **62**, 548–51.

Atal, C. K., Dubey, R. K. and Singh, J. (1985). Biochemical basis of enhanced drug bioavailability by piperine: evidence that piperine is a potent inhibitor of drug metabolism. *J. Pharmacol. Exp. Ther.*, **232**(1), 258–62.

Bano, G., Raina, R. K., Zutshi, U. *et al.* (1991). Effect of piperine on bioavailability and pharmacokinetics of propanolol and theophylline in healthy volunteers. *Eur. J. Clin. Pharmacol.*, **41**, 615–17.

Barnes, J. (1998). Herbal safety high on European phytotherapy agenda. *Inpharma*, **1164**, 20–21.

Blumenthal, M. and Tyler, V. (1997). Herbs and self-medication gain in Germany. *Herbalgram*, **41**, 53.

Blumenthal, M., Busse, W. R., Goldberg, A. *et al.* (1998). *The Complete German Commission E Monographs*. American Botanical Council/Integrative Medicine Communications.

Bos, R., Woerdenbag, H. J., De Smet, P. A. G. M. and Scheffer, J. J. C. (1997). Valeriana species. In *Adverse Effects of Herbal Drugs* (P. A. G. M. De Smet, K. Keller, R. Hänsel and R. F. Chandler, eds.), Vol. 3, pp. 165–180. Springer-Verlag.

Brevoort, P. (1996). The US botanical market, an overview. *Herbalgram*, **36**, 49–57.

Commissie Toetsing Fytotherapeutica (1999). *Inventarisatie en proeftoetsing van plantaardige medicinale bereidingen in Nederland*.

De Smet, P. A. G. M. (1992a). Toxicological outlook on the quality assurance of herbal remedies. In *Adverse Effects of Herbal Drugs* (P. A. G. M. De Smet, K. Keller, R. Hänsel and R. F. Chandler, eds), Vol. 1, pp. 1–72. Springer-Verlag.

De Smet, P. A. G. M. (1992b). Drugs used in non-orthodox medicine. In *Meyler's Side Effects of Drugs*, 12th edn (M. N. G. Dukes, ed.), pp. 1209–32. Elsevier Science Publishers BV.

De Smet, P. A. G. M., Stricker, B. H. C., Wilderink, F. and Wiersinga M. A. (1990). Hyperthyreoidie tijdens het gebruik van kelptabletten. *Ned. T. Geneeskd.*, **134**, 1058–9.

Europam (1998). *Guidelines for Good Agricultural Practice (GAP) of Medicinal and Aromatic Plants*.

European Commission (1998a). Quality of herbal remedies. In *The Rules Governing Medicinal Products in the European Union*, Vol. 3A, pp. 197–202. Office for Official Publications of the European Communities.

European Commission (1998b). Council Directive 75/318/EEC of 20 May 1975 on the approximation of the laws of Member States relating to analytical, pharmacotoxicological and clinical standards and protocols in respect of the testing of medicinal products. In *The Rules Governing Medicinal Products in the European Union*, Vol. 1, pp. 13–40. Office for Official Publications of the European Communities.

European Pharmacopoeia (1989). *Aloes extractum siccum normatum*, 2nd edn. Maisonneuve S.A.

European Scientific Co-operative on Phytotherapy (1997). *Valerianae radix*. Fascicule 4. ESCOP.

Fox, D. W., Hart, M. C., Bergeson, P. S. *et al.* (1978). Pyrrolizidine (Senecio) intoxication mimicking Reye's syndrome. *J. Pediriat.*, **93**, 980–82.

Galizia, E. J. (1983). Clinical curio: hallucinations in elderly tea drinkers. *Br. Med. J.,* **287**, 979.

Grünwald, J. (1995). The European phytomedicines market, figures, trends, analysis. *Herbalgram,* **34**, 60–65.

Hodgson, E. (1987). Measurement of toxicity. In *A Textbook of Modern Toxicology* (E. Hodgson and P. E. Levi, eds), pp. 287–308. Elsevier Science Publishing Co., Inc.

Hori, M., Satoh, S., Maibach, H. I. and Guy, R. H. (1991). Enhancement of propranolol hydrochloride and diazepam skin absorption *in vitro*: effect of enhancer lipophilicity. *J. Pharm. Sci.,* **80**(1), 32–5.

Huxtable, R. J. (1990). The harmful potential of herbal and other plant products. *Drug Safety,* **5**(Suppl. 1), 126–36.

Johnson, A. E., Molyneux, R. J. and Merrill, G. B. (1985). Chemistry of toxic range plants. Variation in pyrrolizidine alkaloid content of Senecio, Amsinckia, and Crotalaria species. *J. Agric. Food Chem.,* **33**, 50–55.

Kumana, C. R., Ng, M., Lin, H. J. *et al.* (1983). Hepatic veno-occlusive disease due to toxic alkaloid in herbal tea. *Lancet,* **2**, 1360–1.

McGuffin, M., Hobbs, C., Upton, R. and Goldberg, A. (1997). *Botanical Safety Handbook.* CRC Press.

Nakayama, K., Fujino, H., Kasai, R. *et al.* (1986). Solubilizing properties of saponins from *Sapindus mukurossi* Gaertn. *Chem. Pharm. Bull.,* **34**(8), 3279–83.

Newall, C. A., Anderson, L. A. and Phillipson, J. D. (1996). *Herbal Medicines, a Guide for Health-care Professionals.* Pharmaceutical Press.

Röder, E. (1982). Nebenwirkungen von Heilpflanzen. *Deutsche Apoth. Ztg.,* **122**(41), 2081–92.

Roitman, J. N. (1981). Comfrey and liver damage. *Lancet,* **1**, 944.

Roth, L., Daunderer, M. and Kormann, K. (1984). *Giftpflanzen, Pflanzengifte.* Ecomed Verlagsgesellschaft.

Roulet, M., Laurini, R., Rivier, L. and Calame, A. (1989). Hepatic veno-occlusive disease in newborn infant of a woman drinking herbal tea. *J. Pedriat.,* **112**(3), 433–6.

Schöpke, T. and Bartlakowski, J. (1997). Effects of saponins on the water solubility of quercetin. *Pharmazie,* **52**, 232–4.

Shoba, G., Joy, D., Joseph, T. *et al.* (1998). Influence of piperine on the pharmacokinetics of curcumin in animals and human volunteers. *Planta Med.,* **64**, 353–6.

Singh, J., Dubey, R. K. and Atal, C. K. (1986). Piperine-mediated inhibition of glucuronidation activity in isolated epithelial cells of the guinea-pig small intestine: evidence that piperine lowers the endogenous UDP-glucuronic acid content. *J. Pharmacol. Exp. Ther.,* **236**(2), 488–93.

Stahl, E. and Keller, K. (1981). Zur Klassifizierung handelsüblicher Kalmusdrogen. *Planta Med.,* **43**, 128–40.

Steinegger, E. and Hänsel, R. (1988). *Lehrbuch der Pharmakognosie und Phytopharmazie.* Springer-Verlag.

Thesen, R. (1988). Phytotherapeutika-nicht immer harmlos. *Pharm. Ztg.,* **133**(1), 38–43.

Vale, S. (1998). Subarachnoid haemorrhage associated with *Ginkgo biloba*.

Lancet, **352**, 36.

Van Beek, T. A., Scheeren, H. A., Rantio, T. *et al.* (1991). Determination of ginkgolides and bilobalide in *Ginkgo biloba* leaves and phytopharmaceuticals. *J. Chromatogr.,* **543**, 375–87.

Van Meer, J. H., Van der Sluis, W. G. and Labadie, R. P. (1977). Onderzoek naar de aanwezigheid van valepotriaten in valeriaanpreparaten. *Pharm. Weekbl.,* **112**, 20–27.

Wagner, H. and Jurcic, K. (1980). In vitro- und in vivo-metabolismus von ^{14}C-didrovaltrate. *Planta Med.,* **38**, 366–76.

Wagner, H., Bladt, S., Daily, A. and Berkulin, W. (1989). *Ginkgo biloba,* DC- und HPLC-Analyse von Ginkgo-Extrakten und Ginkgo-Extrakte enthaltenden Phytopräparaten. *Deutsche Apoth. Ztg.,* **129**(45), 2421–9.

Wichtl, M. (1994). *Herbal Drugs and Phytopharmaceuticals; A Handbook for Practice on a Scientific Basis* (N. G. Bisset, ed., English edition). Medpharm Scientific Publishers.

Williams, A. C. and Barry, B. W. (1991). Terpenes and the lipid-protein-partitioning theory of skin penetration enhancement. *Pharm. Res.,* **8**(1), 17–24.

8

Herbal medicinal products: regulation in the UK and European Union

L. A. Anderson

Introduction

Europe has a long and established tradition in herbal medicines and continues to have the major international market with over 50 per cent of worldwide sales, representing a retail sales volume of over $6 billion (Gruenwald, 1998).

Herbal products are available in all Member States of the European Union, but their importance varies considerably from one country to another and there are differences between Member States in the way herbal products are classified (Deboyser, 1991; Cranz, 1994). A major study undertaken by the AESGP at the request of the European Commission has confirmed this to be the case, and has highlighted the need for clarification of the existing regulatory framework and harmonization of the regulatory requirements to ensure that herbal products have access to the single market for pharmaceuticals (AESGP, 1998).

Different traditions in the therapeutic use of herbal preparations, coupled with different national approaches to their assessment, has resulted in, for example, ginkgo being available as a prescription only medicine in some countries of the EU but as a food supplement in others, and hypericum being accepted as a treatment for depression in some Member States but not in others.

In order for the new European Marketing Authorization procedures for medicinal products to work successfully, efforts have to be made to ensure a harmonized approach to the assessment of safety, quality and efficacy. This remains a challenge for herbal medicinal products, and current European initiatives go some way to identifying the extent of the problem and some possible solutions.

European legislation

According to Council Directive 65/65/EEC (1965), a medicinal product is defined as:

any substance or combination of substances presented for treating or preventing disease in human beings or animals or any substance or combination of substances which may be administered to human beings or animals with a view to making diagnosis or to restoring, correcting or modifying physiological functions in human beings or animals is likewise considered a medicinal product.

Herbal products are considered as medicinal products if they fall within the definition of the Directive. However, the legal classification is complicated by the fact that in most Member States herbal products are available both as medicinal products with therapeutic claims and also as food/dietary supplements without medicinal claims. The situation is further complicated in that some Member States, including the UK, have national provisions which permit certain herbal medicinal products to be exempt from the licensing provisions under specific conditions.

Council Directive 65/65/EEC requires that, in order to obtain a marketing authorization for a medicinal product, proof of quality, safety and efficacy must be presented. The specific requirements for the dossier and expert reports are laid down in Council Directive 75/318/EEC (1975), as amended by Directive 91/507/EEC (1991). In addition to the requirements of the Directives, specific notes for guidance are available from the Committee on Proprietary Medicinal Products (CPMP), which provides advice to applicants on particular aspects. Two CPMP guidelines are currently available on herbal medicinal products dealing with aspects of quality and manufacture (Quality of Herbal Medicinal Products, 1989; Manufacture of Herbal Medicinal Products, 1997).

There are no specific guidelines on safety and efficacy requirements for herbal medicinal products, and it is these areas that present the greatest divergence in approach between Member States. Many applicants rely on published data to support their applications, so-called 'bibliographic applications', and Member States have adopted different approaches depending on the traditional use of the herbal product in their country.

UK position

In the UK, medicines legislation requires all medicines to be authorized (licensed) before being placed on the market, unless exempted from that requirement. Products sold or supplied for human use as medicinal products are controlled under the Medicines for Human Use (Marketing Authorisations Etc.) Regulations 1994 SI 3144 and the Medicines Act 1968, and are regulated by the Medicines Control Agency (MCA) (Statutory Instrument, 1994; The Medicines Act 1968).

The Medicines for Human Use (Marketing Authorisations Etc.) Regulations 1994 took effect in January 1995, and effectively implemented the full range of controls set out in Directive 65/65/ EEC which apply to 'relevant medicinal products' as defined in the Regulations. The main controls include application requirements and procedures for the grant, variation and renewal of UK licences, requirements in relation to pharmacovigilance, labelling and package leaflets as well as provisions for suspension, compulsory variation or revocation and related enforcement issues. The Medicines Act 1968, and secondary legislation made under it, remains the legal basis for other aspects of medicines control, including manufacturers' and wholesale dealers' authorizations, controls on sale and supply and controls on promotion.

Herbal products are available through various retail outlets such as pharmacies, healthfood shops, supermarkets and departmental stores. These products fall into three main categories:

1. Licensed herbal medicinal products
2. Herbal remedies exempt from licensing
3. Food supplements.

The majority of herbal products are marketed without medicinal claims and are available either as food supplements or as herbal remedies exempt from licensing. When medicinal claims are made, the product is always subject to licensing. The distinction, however, between products sold as food supplements and those sold as exempt herbal remedies is a grey area because of uncertainties and difficulties in defining the status of products occupying the borderline between medicines and foods.

Herbal products supplied as food supplements are controlled under food legislation by the Ministry of Agriculture, Fisheries and Foods (MAFF). Herbal remedies exempt from licensing are controlled under the Medicines Act 1968, and are the responsibility of the MCA.

Licensed herbal products

Herbal medicinal products sold with therapeutic claims are subject to the licensing provisions and are required to hold product licences (marketing authorizations), and manufacturers are subject to inspection and compliance with Good Manufacturing Practice

(GMP) (1997). Currently herbal medicinal products are assessed in line with European legislation, and applications for herbal products are handled in the same way as other medicinal products. The use of the 'traditional herbal remedy' approach, which was adopted for the review of herbal remedies (see below), is no longer applied.

Where an applicant seeks to license a herbal product and the active ingredient(s) is not currently licensed in the UK, the product falls within the 'new active substance' category and a full dossier is required in accordance with Directive 75/318/EEC.

Where the herbal ingredients are already used in UK licensed products, applications can be submitted under the abridged procedure. If the proposed indications are already approved for a given herbal ingredient, the applicant will normally refer to published data to support the safety and efficacy aspects of the application. If an applicant proposes a new indication, route of administration or patient population, the application will be considered as a 'complex' abridged application and appropriate clinical and toxicological data will be required to support the proposed use. In all cases a full pharmaceutical dossier is required relating to the formulation proposed for marketing.

The majority of licensed herbal medicinal products available in the UK, of which there are approximately 500, have been on the market for some considerable time. Most products originally held Product Licences of Right (PLRs), and these were automatically granted to products already on the market when the Medicines Act came into force in the early 1970s (see Review of herbal remedies below).

Most of the herbal ingredients used in licensed herbal medicines have been used as traditional remedies for centuries without major safety problems, and the majority are included in the General Sales List (The Medicines (Products other than Veterinary Drugs) General Sales List, 1944). Potentially hazardous plants such as digitalis, rauwolfia and strychnos are specifically controlled under the Medicines Act as prescription only medicines (POM), and thus are not available other than via a registered medical practitioner (The Medicines (Products other than Veterinary Drugs) Prescription Only Order, 1983).

Herbal remedies exempt from licensing

Under the Medicines Act (Statutory Instrument, 1971), herbal remedies

  manufactured and sold or supplied in accordance with specific exemptions set out in Section 12(1) or (2) or Article 2 of the

Medicines (Exemptions from Licences) (Special and Transitional Cases) Order 1971 (SI 1450) are exempt from the requirement to hold product licences.

Section 12 of the Medicines Act allows exemption from licensing for herbal remedies sold or supplied in very specific circumstances. The exempt products are those supplied by herbalists to individual patients on the recommendation of the practitioner. Also exempt are products consisting solely of dried, crushed or comminuted herbs, and those made by a holder of a Special Manufacturing Licence on behalf of a herbalist. In all cases, the exempt products are supplied without written recommendations as to their use.

The exemptions are intended to give herbal practitioners the flexibility they need to prepare their own remedies for individual patients without the burden of licensing and to enable simple dried herbs to be readily available to the public.

As long as the product concerned is a herbal remedy made from simple processes, a shopkeeper (i.e. not necessarily a pharmacist) may sell or supply against the prescription of an approved practitioner, unless the POM order specifies to the contrary.

In addition, other herbal ingredients are controlled under The Medicines (Retail Sale or Supply of Herbal Remedies) Order 1977 SI 2130. This order specifies 25 plants that cannot be supplied except through pharmacies, and includes well-known toxic plants such as areca, crotalaria, dryopteris and strophanthus. The order also specifies a number of potent plant species which can be supplied by herbal practitioners, such as Aconite species, belladonna, ephedra and hyoscyamus, but the doses and routes of administration are restricted.

Review of herbal remedies in the UK

The majority of licensed herbal medicinal products available in the UK have been on the market for some considerable time. Most products originally held Product Licences of Right (PLRs) and these were granted automatically to products already on the market when the Medicines Act came into force in the early 1970s.

In order to be issued with PLRs for their products, pharmaceutical companies had simply to provide details of the products and evidence that the products had been marketed prior to 1971; no scientific assessment was undertaken. This procedure applied to all medicinal products, including herbal remedies, and in total some 39 000 PLRs were granted. It was obvious that at some future date all PLR products (including herbal remedies) would have to be assessed by the Licensing Authority (LA) for their quality, safety and efficacy, in the same manner as those products that had applied for a product licence after 1971. European Community (EC) legislation required that this review of all PLR products be completed by May 1990.

During the review of herbal remedies, the Licensing Authority on the advice of its Advisory Bodies agreed to adopt a pragmatic approach to the assessment and accept bibliographic evidence of safety and efficacy, provided the product was intended for minor self-limiting conditions. No evidence was required from new clinical trials, provided the manufacturer labelled the product as a 'traditional herbal remedy for the symptomatic relief of...' and included 'if symptoms persist consult your doctor'.

The Licensing Authority was not, however, prepared to relax the requirements for proof of efficacy for products indicated for more serious indications such as hypertension. Thus, evidence was required from controlled clinical trials for herbal remedies indicated for conditions considered to be inappropriate for self-diagnosis and treatment.

In its assessment of the safety of herbal remedies, the Licensing Authority agreed to rely as far as possible on the work of other agencies. Thus, supporting evidence of safety, for example, included acceptance of a herbal ingredient for food use or inclusion of a herbal ingredient on Schedule I of the General Sales List.

Herbal medicinal products in other European Member States

National procedures implemented by Member States to comply with the earlier EC requirements to review all licensed herbal products by May 1990 have differed from state to state, as a herbal remedy may have a well-established use in one country but not in another. Clearly European harmonization on what is acceptable for the assessment of quality, safety and efficacy for these products is required to enable the mutual recognition system to operate.

New European marketing authorization procedures

The legal classification of herbal remedies within Europe and the problems involved in harmonizing their assessment have been reviewed (Deboyser, 1991; Cranz, 1994; Keller, 1994). The advent of the new pan-European marketing authorization system that came into operation in 1995 has raised a number of questions about herbal remedies and their possible access to other European markets. The new systems for marketing authorizations involve three procedures: centralized, decentralized (mutual recognition) and national.

The centralized procedure is mandatory for biotechnology products and optional for high-technology products and medicinal products containing new active substances. The decentralized procedure or mutual recognition system involves agreement of assessment between the Member States involved, and was optional until 1 January 1998 for products requesting authorization in more than one Member State. The current situation allows for simultaneous national applications, but the mutual recognition system will automatically be involved once an authorization has been granted in the first Member State. Existing national procedures will remain for medicinal products requesting authorization in a single Member State only. In addition, the European Commission have agreed that national procedures can continue for bibliographic application.

Experience with the mutual recognition procedure

To date, experience of herbal medicinal products within mutual recognition procedures has been limited. There has been some reluctance on behalf of the industry, but a few single component products have gone through successfully, namely, valerian, ispaghula.

ESCOP

An important initiative in the harmonization process has been the formation of ESCOP (European Scientific Cooperative for Phyto-therapy), an umbrella organization representing national associations for phytotherapy. Since 1990, ESCOP has produced a series of monographs on herbal drugs drawn from published scientific literature and experience of national delegates (ESCOP, 1996). A number of the ESCOP monographs (frangula bark, senna fruit, senna leaf) have been adopted by the European CPMP (Committee on Proprietary Medicinal Products) as core-SPCs (Summary of Product Characteristics) for herbal medicinal products.

Ad Hoc Working Group on Herbal Medicinal Products

In 1997, the *Ad Hoc* Working Group on Herbal Medicinal Products was established by the European Commission, the European

Medicines Evaluation Agency (EMEA) Executive Director and the EMEA Management Board. This Working Group is made up of representatives from the Member States, the European Parliament, the European Commission and the European Pharmacopoeia. The Working Group has carried out a comprehensive review of existing guidelines, and has updated/adapted them to the particular needs of herbal medicinal products.

AESGP study on herbal medicinal products in the EU

The AESGP has just completed a major study on behalf of the European Commission into herbal medicinal products within the EU (AESGP, 1998). The main objectives have been to clarify the current legal position in each Member State, compare actual practices in the assessment of safety, quality and efficacy, evaluate possible divergences in the legal position or the assessment criteria and make recommendations on how best to safeguard public health while allowing free movement of herbal medicinal products throughout the Community.

The study has confirmed that there are problems with divergent approaches within Member States and has concluded that in order to ensure a harmonized approach, clarification is needed as to the requirements detailed in Directive 75/318/EEC.

Future perspectives

The European Commission intends to put forward proposals to clarify the data requirements for applicants when seeking a licence for 'well established medicinal products', and this would include herbal remedies. Any proposed changes would probably be achieved by amendments to the Annex to Directive 75/318/EEC. The proposals will need to be considered in detail by Member States, but they may go some way to clarifying the regulatory position for herbal medicinal products in the EU.

References

AESGP (1998). *Herbal Medicinal Products in the UK*. The Association of the European Self-Medication Industry.
Council Directive 65/65/EEC. (1965).
Council Directive 75/318/EEC. (1975).
Council Directive 91/507/EEC. (1991).

Cranz, H. (1994). Medicinal plants and phytomedicines within the European Community. *Herbalgram,* **30**, 50–53.

Deboyser, P. (1991). Traditional herbal remedies around the globe and modern perspectives. *Swiss Pharma.,* **13**, 86–9.

ESCOP (1996). *Monographs on the Medicinal Uses of Plant Drugs.* European Scientific Co-operative on Phytotherapy.

Good Manufacturing Practices (1997). *The Rules Governing Medicinal Products in the European Community,* Vol 4. Office for Official Publications of the European Community.

Gruenwald, J. (1998). The emerging role of herbal medicine in health care in Europe. *Drug Inf. J.,* **32**, 151–3.

Keller, K. (1994). Phytotherapy on the European level. *Eur. Phytotelegram,* **6**, 40–49.

Manufacture of Herbal Medicinal Products (1997). *The Rules Governing Medicinal Products in the European Community,* Vol. 4, 99–101. Office for Official Publications of the European Community.

Quality of Herbal Medicinal Products (1989). *The Rules Governing Medicinal Products in the European Community,* Vol. 3, 31–7. Office for Official Publications of the European Community.

Statutory Instrument (1971) 1450. The Medicines (Exemptions from Licences) (Special and Transitional Cases) Order.

Statutory Instrument (1977) 2130. The Medicines (Retail Sale or Supply of Herbal Remedies) Order.

Statutory Instrument (1994) 3144. The Medicines for Human Use (Marketing Authorizations Etc) Regulations.

The Medicines Act 1968. HMSO.

The Medicines (Products other than Veterinary Drugs) General Sales List, SI No. 769 (1984) as amended SI No.1540 (1985); SI No. 1129 (1990); SI No. 2410 (1994).

The Medicines (Products Other than Veterinary Drugs) (Prescription Only) Order (1983).

Conclusion

E. Ernst

Both the sales figures for herbal remedies and the uptake of medical herbalism by the population speak for themselves: plant-based medicines are an undeniable reality and the medical professions have to face this reality, regardless of whether they are proponents or opponents. This book is an attempt to guide those interested in the subject safely through the maze.

Medical herbalism thrives on its long and diverse traditions. Chapter 1 represents an attempt to bridge the gap between this ancient history and the recent scientific evaluation of phytomedicine. The focus here is on herbal drugs acting on the central nervous system. Rosemary, sage, melissa, ginkgo, ginseng and St John's wort are used as examples. The authors make it clear that safe and effective therapies have emerged and are continuing to emerge from the archives of ethnopharmacology. The careful and intelligent synthesis of traditional knowledge with modern scientific phyto-pharmacological evidence shows us an effective way forward.

Chapter 2 provides valuable details on prevalence and sales figures in various countries. This confirms the widespread use of herbal remedies and points to important national differences. This chapter also explores the reasons why so many people turn towards herbal remedies. At least in part, these reasons constitute a serious criticism of orthodox medicine. The behaviour of consumers is discussed in relation to over-the-counter herbal and synthetic medicines, and important differences are pointed out. These differences are relevant not least to pharmacists. The attitudes of pharmacists, who are often the only healthcare professionals at the interface with the consumer, towards plant-based therapies are explored.

Chapter 3 defines new targets for phytopharmacological research. A stepwise approach consisting of the isolation of the major active constituents of plants, their structural clarification, chemical and biological standardization, elucidation of pharmacological effects and determination of clinical efficacy through clinical trials is suggested. Wagner advocates investigating individual parts of a complex system in order to arrive at an understanding of the system as a whole. The examples provided relate to hawthorn, stinging nettle and garlic. He argues that understanding the mechanisms of action of phytomedicines is a crucial precondition for any rational clinical use of such drugs. Moreover, he points out that our knowledge is incomplete in many of these areas. This also applies to defining adequate dosages and long-term effects.

The concept that particular plant constituents act synergistically is deeply imbedded in the traditions of various ethnic forms of traditional herbalism. The whole plant, it is argued, almost by definition constitutes a better and more holistic treatment than therapy with one or more isolated active ingredients. In Chapter 4, Williamson critically evaluates the evidence for or against this concept. She describes the amazing paucity of hard data in this area and the inadequacy of sound methodologies to evaluate the problem. After defining what synergy and antagonism mean, she continues to differentiate between polyvalent action, synergy in single herb extracts and synergy in multi-herb preparations. The latter is, of course, particularly important for various forms of traditional herbalism such as traditional Chinese medicine or Ayurveda. Williamson concludes that synergy does exist, and provides examples where the phenomenon has been demonstrated beyond reasonable doubt, e.g. ginkgo and St John's wort.

Chapter 5 addresses some of the most crucial issues related to quality and standardization of herbal medicines. Loew and Schroedter point out that quality is determined by all steps in the production process of herbal products. This involves the agricultural aspects such as soil, climate, fertilization, pesticide and herbicide use and seed quality, as well as harvesting techniques. It also includes the processing of the plant or part of plant and, of course, the manufacturing and standardization processes as well as the analytical methodology of quality control. It is clear that the quality of a herbal product is a prime determinant of both its efficacy and safety.

Chapter 6 represents an attempt to summarize concisely our present knowledge related to efficacy. Rather than relying on single trials, of which we have many (too many to be detailed here) and which can (and frequently do) contradict each other in terms of outcome, this chapter relies on systematic reviews of controlled clinical trials. Such analyses are now available for an increasing number of phytomedicines: aloe vera, artichoke, feverfew, ginger, ginkgo, ginseng, horse chestnut, kava, peppermint, St John's wort and valerian are all dealt with in this chapter. As expected, the results of these systematic reviews and meta-analyses are variable and not devoid of surprises. For some herbal medicines the evidence for efficacy is relatively sound, e.g. St John's wort or kava; however, there are other popular herbal remedies where this is not the case, e.g. ginseng or valerian. There could be more than one explanation. For instance, the clinical trials might be too sparse or methodologically flawed so that firm conclusions are not permissible. Alternatively, the herbal remedy might simply not be sufficiently efficacious to generate a positive overall result. At the very least, this chapter shows that systematic reviews and meta-analyses of phytomedicines can provide valuable answers. Therefore, more such evidence should be generated. Reviews and meta-analyses are not, however, without limitations, and have to be interpreted with care, particularly in view of the danger of false negative results.

In Chapter 7, Halkes takes on the task of tackling the important safety issues related to herbal medicines. Consumers of plant-based treatments are all too often led to believe that 'natural' can be equated with 'harmless'. This is unfortunately not necessarily the case. The safety issues are complex, and range from direct toxicity of the medicinal plant to the possibility of interactions with synthetic drugs and to contamination or adulteration of botanical drugs. Halkes constructively points us to a way of minimizing risks in the future through instituting several layers of safety measures. The chapter concludes by providing useful concrete data from a Dutch survey related to the safety of herbal remedies.

In Chapter 8, Anderson completes this book by providing an authoritative update on the regulation of herbal medicinal products in the UK and EU. In the area of phytomedicine regulatory problems abound, and with some regularity they come to the attention of the public. Whenever this happens they are then fiercely debated. There are many interests at stake, and the involvement of monetary interests does not usually enhance clarity. Anderson details all relevant issues as they pertain to licensed herbal products and those remedies that are exempt from licensing. She also gives valuable information about the most important regulatory bodies in Europe and their respective roles. The message that emerges is that regulation of herbal medicines is not an end in its own; neither is it a means of unnecessary control by 'the establishment'. Its prime aim is to minimize the risk for users of herbal products. Therefore, the quality of herbal regulations will have to be measured by the degree to which consumer safety is achieved.

This book cannot cover all aspects of medical herbalism. It is meant as a concise introduction to some of the most important aspects. All chapters are extensively referenced, and thus encourage the reader to explore particular interests further. The book as a whole shows quite clearly, I believe, that an evolution has taken place during the last decades with the gradual maturation of traditional herbalism into evidence-based phytotherapy. This process is by no means complete, but important steps have been taken and new evidence has been generated at all levels of inquiry. In the past, this type of knowledge and discussion has often been restricted to German-speaking audiences – much of the evidence was generated in Germany and published in German, often in journals not referenced in standard databases. I hope that this book renders it more accessible, particularly to English-speaking audiences. I am confident that it will be a useful text for all healthcare professionals with a serious interest in medical herbalism.

Bibliography

Bensoussan, A. and Myers, S. P. (1996). *Towards a Safer Choice: The Practice of Traditional Chinese Medicine in Australia.* Victoria: MacArthur.

Blumenthal, M., Busse, W. R., Goldberg, A. *et al.* (1998). *The Complete German Commission E Monographs.* Boston: American Botanical Council/Integrative Medicine Communications.

British Herbal Pharmacopoeia (1996) (4th edn). Exeter: British Herbal Medicine Association.

Eldin, S. and Dunford, A. (1999). *Herbal Medicine in Primary Care.* Oxford: Butterworth-Heinemann.

Eskinazi, D., Blumenthal, M., Farnsworth, N. and Riggins, C. W. (1999). *Botanical Medicine Efficacy, Quality Assurance and Regulation.* New York: Mary Ann Liebert Inc.

Harborne, J. B., Baxter, H. and Moss, G. P. (1996). *Dictionary of Plant Toxins.* Chichester: John Wiley & Sons Ltd.

Jonas, W. B. and Levin J. S. (1999). *Essentials of Complementary and Alternative Medicine.* Canada: Lippincott Williams & Wilkins.

Kanba, S. and Richelson, E. (1999). *Herbal Medicines for Neuropsychiatric Diseases: Current Developments and Research.* Tokyo: Seiwa Shoten Publishers.

Miller, L. G. and Murray, W. J. (1998). *Herbal Medicinals: A Clinician's Guide.* New York: The Haworth Press Inc.

Newall, C. A., Anderson, L. A. and Phillipson, J. D. (1996). *Herbal Medicines: A Guide for Health-care Professionals.* London: The Pharmaceutical Press.

Robbers, J. E. and Tyler, V. E. (1999). *Tyler's Herbs of Choice. The Therapeutic Use of Phytomedicinals.* New York: The Haworth Press Inc.

Ross, I. A. (1999). *Medicinal Plants of the World. Chemical Constituents, Traditional and Modern Medicinal Uses.* New Jersey: Human Press Inc.

Schulz, V., Hänsel, R. and Tyler, V. E. (1998). *Rational Phytotherapy: A Physician's Guide to Herbal Medicine.* Berlin: Springer-Verlag.

Index